GOK WAN

How to Look Good Naked

FROM THE HIT TV SERIES

HarperCollinsPublishers

To all of my wonderful family, whom I love more
than any one book could tell them: Daddy, Mummy,
Oilen, Kwoklyn, Lisa, Maya Lily, Lola Rose and my
ever beautiful Nanny Nash.

HarperCollins*Publishers*
77–85 Fulham Palace Road
Hammersmith, London W6 8JB

The HarperCollins website address is: www.harpercollins.co.uk

First published in 2007 by HarperCollins*Publishers*
This edition 2008

10 9 8 7 6 5 4 3 2

© Gok Wan 2007

Gok Wan asserts the moral right to be
identified as the author of this work

Edited by Angela Buttolph

Studio photography © Mike Owen
Studio photography digital processing by Nick Pearce at Reflection Digital
Reportage photography © David Leahy

A catalogue record of this book is
available from the British Library

ISBN-13 978-0-00-726724-8
ISBN-10 0-00-726724-X

Printed and bound in Italy
by L.E.G.O SpA

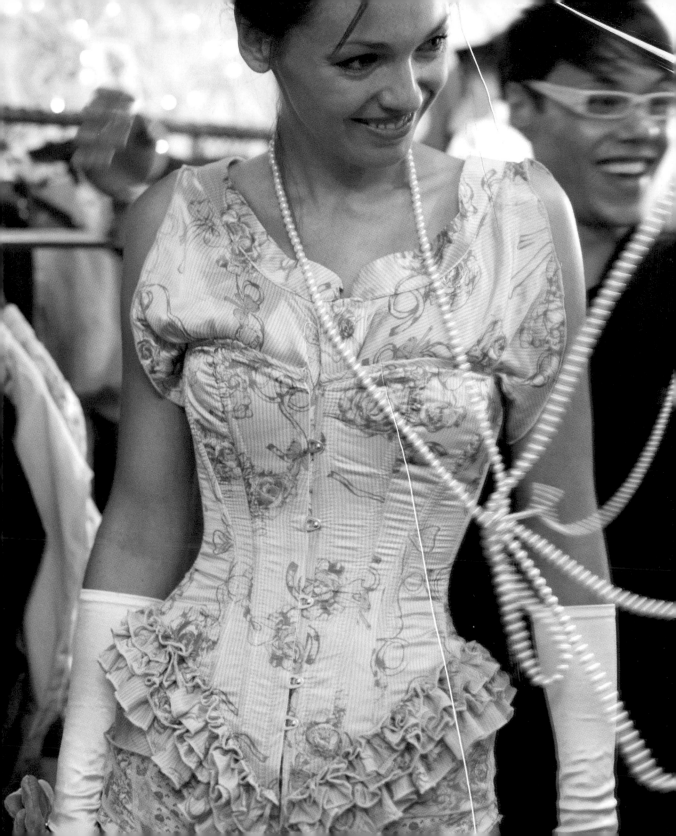

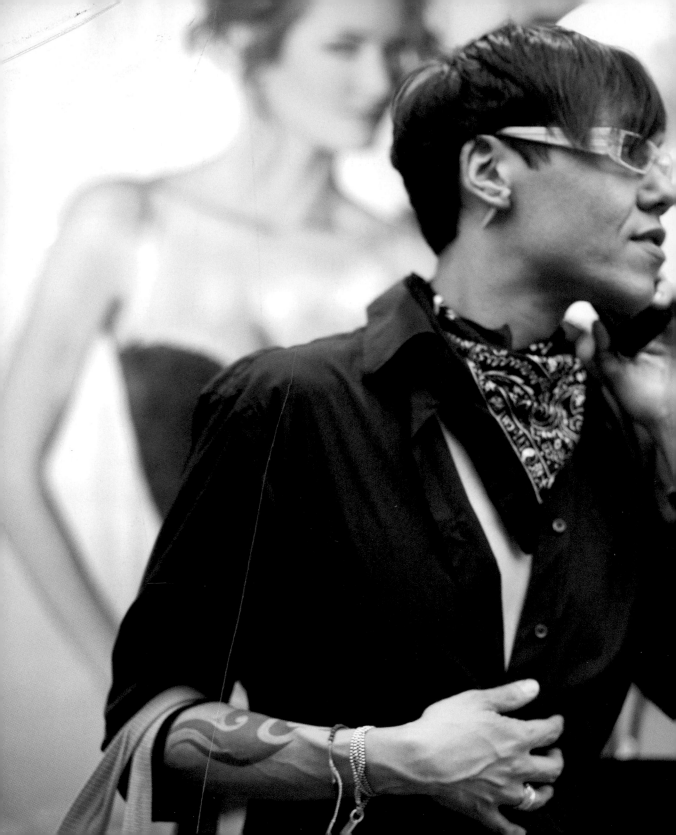

Introduction

use your look, gorgeous girl

Take a look at what you're wearing right now, and if your outfit doesn't say, 'I'm the Most Gorgeous Creature Who Ever Lived', keep reading.

The way you dress tells the whole world how you feel about your body. And what you wear influences how good you feel about yourself. It's that feeling you get when you put on your favourite pair of jeans – you just know that cute ass of yours will turn heads.

This is the effect that everything in your wardrobe should have. You deserve to feel fabulous all day, every day. And this, my sweet, is how I'm going to help you.

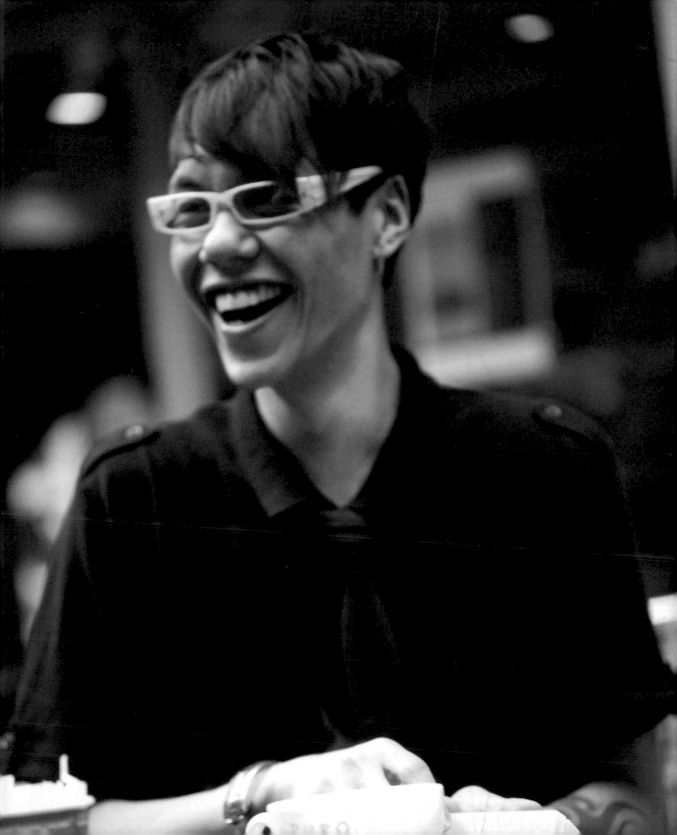

Stop Judging, Start Loving

Some lucky girls love every inch of their bodies. Maybe that's you. Maybe you can't wait to strip off: in bed with your partner, on a crowded beach, in those communal changing rooms most of us hate. Maybe you're even reading this book naked (in which case, I really hope you've taken it home first!).

As for the rest of us, we aren't quite so lucky. Too many of us often feel insecure about our bodies. I would love it if everybody everywhere felt good about themselves, but, sadly, we don't. We need to be reminded that our bodies are amazing things of natural beauty. We should feel proud to inhabit them! In some ways it's not that surprising. We're exposed to three thousand images of models and celebrities in the average week: looking skinny, preened, and perfect (don't you just hate them?).

I've worked in fashion for ten years, first as a hair and make up artist, then as a stylist. I love my job! I love the glamour of it all. Every morning I wake up and I am always excited to be working with such talented people.

But believe me, a lot of hard work goes into making each beautiful image: from hours of hair and make-up, to fabulously flattering lighting, expert photography and careful and creative computer-editing of the pictures afterwards. There is a reason why it takes a whole day, and a team of twelve, to shoot five or six images for a fashion magazine! (And therefore why all those spur-of-the-moment snaps of you are never quite as flattering.) And yet we compare ourselves with all these unrealistic images of perfection, even though many of the photos we see have been stretched, retouched and airbrushed.

So why compare ourselves when what we see isn't real? It's time for real women to fight back!

Women want to look good – but for real! And, in reality, women come in all shapes and sizes. You're a real woman, so you do have curves and lumps and bumps, asymmetrical breasts and stretch marks. And you know what? That's okay – it's normal, and it's fine. Your body is naturally beautiful and you should be celebrating that.

One of the hardest parts on *How to Look Good Naked* was what I call the Mirror Moment. In order to transform each of my gorgeous girls, I had to see exactly what I was working with. But to do that I had to get them to strip off in front of the mirror, and to face their fears. Let me tell you, it was really heartbreaking to see women breaking down at having to look at their own reflections, sometimes for the first time in years. It was hard for these women to look at themselves because they had really tried to be invisible for so long. As a result, they were losing certain parts of their lives: relationships with their partners or their children, or the confidence to do certain things, from going on holiday (to avoid stripping off on the beach) to going shopping (to avoid those communal changing rooms).

Nearly all of them seemed to be saying, 'I can't do this any more. I've been afraid for so many years to ask for help, and I haven't known where to turn for it.'

I'm going to be your helping hand. On the show, I have to be confidant, best friend, security blanket, shoulder to cry on, expert and judge: quite a tall order, but I loved it! I'll be doing that for you in this book, too. In only four weeks we transformed my Gokettes; getting them back in tune with their bodies, and their partners. And I can do that for you, too.

You are absolutely not on your own. Nine out of ten British women say they hate everything about their bodies. But now it's time to stop wanting to be invisible, or hiding in schlumpy clothes, or turning the light out in the bedroom, or avoiding going shopping. Come on, ladies, let's see you strut your stuff!

Work That Look, Girl!

Everyone needs an image, whether it's for a job interview or a date. On photo-shoots I basically work with very creative, controlled images for some of the world's biggest celebrities.

The first life-changing makeover I ever did was on myself. I was bullied when I was younger for being fat. Back then, I was really overweight (seriously: they used to call me Hubba Blubba). I've always had a big mouth, so I could hold my own. But then one summer, when I was about twelve, I suddenly decided enough was enough. At that time I was living in a pair of elasticated-waist tracksuit bottoms from M&S. I'd like to tell you I was an early pioneer of the funky sportswear-chic look, but really they were the only clothes that fitted apart from a tent!

My transformation started with a sharp new haircut, all gelled into place. Then I got my mum to take me shopping (at Next!), and I bought beige chinos, brown brogues, a cream Arran jumper and a beige checked shirt. I was so neutral and beige, I looked like an artificial limb. (Before you doubt my fashion credentials and throw this book out of the window, can I just say that it was actually quite cool way back then, I promise – prosthetic chic!)

I didn't lose any weight that summer, but when I went back to school in the autumn, no one shouted at me any more. I was way too cool for that school! The only difference was I'd stopped hiding away in my tracksuit bottoms. I stood big, bold and oh, so beautiful. I had started to Use My Look, and I never looked back.

In fact, I didn't properly lose weight until I was much older. But even today, I still use different looks to show the different personalities of Gok: skater boy, rock star, sharp-suited player. So, from a very early age, fashion has always been very important to me – almost like my armour.

That's what I wanted to do on *How to Look Good Naked*. I wanted to teach people the secrets of how to feel good about themselves. Women learn the rules of what suits them, and then stick to them. And it shows.

In this book I'm going to give you a shopping list for the best shapes to suit you. Think of it as a blueprint for your signature style. As you'll see, I've singled out eight luscious body shapes and the most insanely flattering styles to go with them. Expect plenty of what I call Best Friend Honesty: me telling you what you need to hear, in a nice way (I love my girls!).

One of the body shapes should fit you as perfectly as a Jimmy Choo. But don't feel you have to limit yourself strictly to that chapter alone — a girl's entitled to more than one perfect pair of shoes! Let's say you're a juicy pear-shaped girl. *Juicy girl* is the natural chapter for you, no doubt about it. Another priority for you though is making the most of your tush, so take a good long look at *Booty babe*. I want you shaking your cute ass with pride!

Whatever your shape, make sure you dive undercover to the underwear chapter on p. 155. Lingerie can make or break an outfit, so even if you follow Gok's shop-for-your-shape advice to the letter, you ain't gonna look half as hot with the wrong underwear.

Above all though, I want you to use what you've got, and learn to love it, work it and flaunt it. So even if you'd like to lose a bit of weight (although you look pretty good to me), I'm not going to start talking about dieting. I want to show you how to work with what you've got RIGHT NOW; to make yourself look amazing RIGHT NOW. Don't think you have to wait to lose weight before improving how you look and feel. This book is not about being mean to yourself or hiding that gorgeous body of yours. I want you to start thinking positively about yourself. NOW. The world is ready for you and you need to be ready for it.

Make Fashion Work For You

Whilst we're on the subject of reinvention, let's make another thing **clear. I love the** idea of reinvention – I think it's such a beautiful thing **that any human** being can do it. But let's say No to the knife. I really **believe women** should not be forced to think that plastic surgery is the **only option for** improving their looks. I would much rather you threw **away an unflatt**ering skirt that makes you look fat than have ten pounds **of fat sucked ou**t of your thighs.

Everybody has bits of their body they don't like, but other people **rarely view your** body in the same way that you do. I think that was one **of the most im**portant lessons my girls learned on the show. All of them **had different** areas of their body that they hated: their 'love handles', **their 'saddl**e bags', their 'bingo wings'. But when we polled the public **(showing** them naughty projections of my naked Gokettes!) the feed-**back was** always so positive. There's a lesson here that we'll come back **to later.**

So I'm going to show you how to transform yourself without having **to nip**, tuck, crunch or starve. Believe me: the right clothes can RADI-**CAL**LY change the way you look and they're cheaper, more effective **and** infinitely more pleasurable than surgery! Besides, shopping is the **ult**imate cardio workout – it's the best exercise. I lost two pounds in last **y**ear's Selfridges sale!

I also want you to think about quality over quantity. In the show I take all my girls to high-street stores. I also use high-street clothes on photo shoots, so you know Gok's no label snob! On the other hand, my years in fashion have taught me that it's better to buy one great coat (in the perfect, most insanely flattering shade and shape) that you will wear for years, than to buy a few so-so jackets just because they're bargains or this week's hot look.

Keep your eye on the long-term game. I would recommend you buy even just one high-quality classic piece a season: a beautiful white shirt, say, or an elegant little black dress, or the perfect trench coat, to build up a gorgeous wardrobe over time. Timeless classics will save your ass in the future when you're having a dilemma day.

So this is your reference book: somewhere you can go back to for a little bit of security, a little bit of community, to get some tips, to get lost in some beautiful pictures and to get inspired by the amazing world that is fashion – which has probably seemed like your worst enemy for so long. This is a little bit of fashion and glamour just for you.

It's about making fashion work for you.

What I want you to do from this moment onwards is to begin appreciating your body and start saying thank you to yourself for being you. I want you to take a long, hard look at yourself, and at what you have been trying to cover up – a beautiful body that you should be proud to live in! By the end of the book you will be shopping again, shagging again, and you will be able to look in the mirror and really love what you see.

So you've got it, and now it's time to flaunt it! Yeah, baby!

Now turn the page. Honey, let's go forth and conquer...

Juicy Girl...

pear-shaped but oh so juicy

Sixty per cent of British women are pear-shaped.
That's almost two-thirds of the population (18 million). You are the classic English rose, my gorgeous!

There is something so graceful about the pear-
shaped silhouette – from the delicate femininity of
your shoulders and waist, to the womanly sensuality of your hips.

Honey, you've got it all going on!

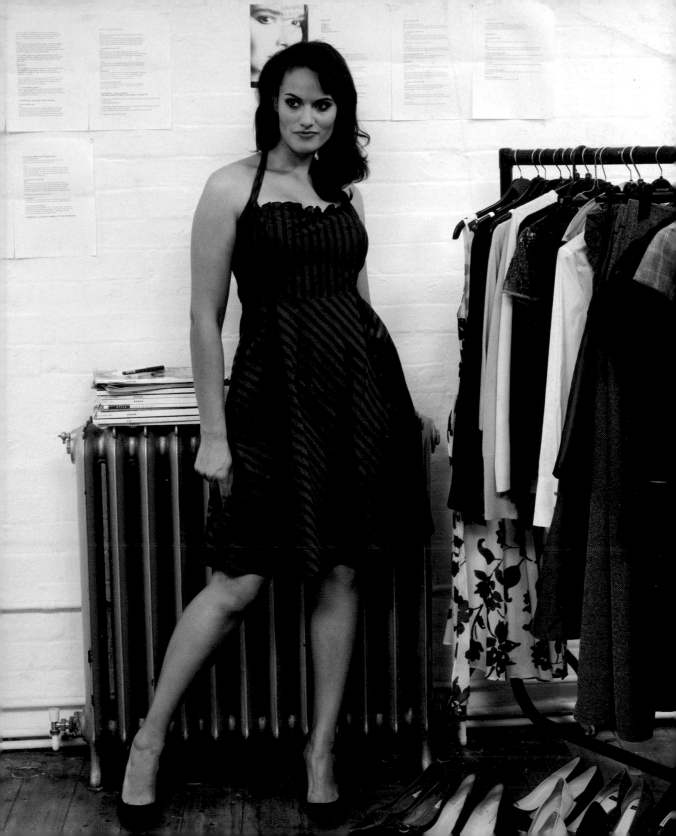

Your Magic Fashion Formula

- Skim the hips to slim the width, with A-line skirts and loose trousers.

- Broaden the shoulders with structured tops and jackets.

Artists, photographers and sculptors have been obsessed by your shape for centuries: from Modigliani's nude portraits of reclining pear-shaped beauties, to the photographer Man Ray, whose saucy depiction of the female body as a voluptuous violin was considered pretty risqué at the time.

So why do half of the British pears hate their shape?

I often see hippy chicks trying to cover up their beautiful bottom in engulfing baggy trousers, while over-emphasizing the slimmest part of their body with a tiny skin-tight T-shirt. Okay, I get what they're doing, but this just throws the perfect curves of a pear-shaped body totally out of whack.

Today, women such as Britney Spears, Jennifer Love Hewitt, Mischa Barton, and *Sex and the City*'s Kristin Davis are all pear-shaped style icons who have worked out how to play up their proportions. For starters, a key part of your wardrobe should be a push-up bra. Boosting your boobs will give balance to your body (see Underwear section).

Your shape is great, but, like a juicy pear, it needs to be handled with care. So here are some tips for clever dressing.

Juicy Girl's Perfect Skirts

A slight A-line skirt in a stiff fabric such as denim, thick cotton, leather, etc. will echo and streamline your curves. Volume on a skirt de-emphasizes the width of your hips. Wearing your hemline just below the knee will emphasize your slim ankles and calves.

STEP AWAY FROM THE RAIL:

- Everyone gets jealous of pear-shaped women's flat stomachs (grrr). Wearing skirts with pleats or that gather from the waistband will just add bulk where there isn't any, so stick to flat-fronted A-line styles.

- Avoid skirts in shiny fabrics such as satin, taffeta, or with sequins, etc., which all make the area appear larger.

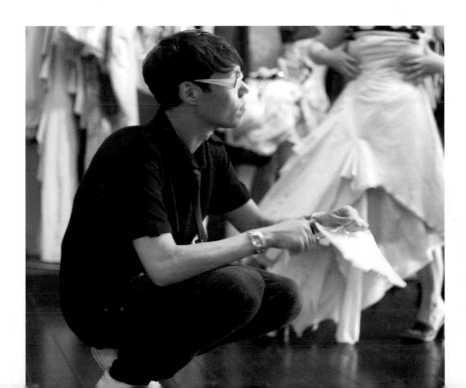

Juicy Girl's Perfect Dresses

Let's face it, your body is custom-made. You're not an average, production-line, off-the-rack kind of woman. There are plenty of girls out there who are a bog-standard size 14, or a spot-on size medium, or whatever. But your gorgeous body is a little more high maintenance, which I love (I'm all about high maintenance). What I'm trying to say is that you need a dress that works for you, not the other way round.

Crossover styles are great, because the straight horizontal line of the hem is disrupted, which de-emphasizes any broadness in this area (asymmetrical or handkerchief hems are also good for this reason). A large all-over pattern (the more random the better) is the best optical illusion to stop your top looking too teeny. For those with smaller shoulders, a halter-neck dress will broaden your top half and balance you out – it's all about balance, sweet cheeks!

One of the best styles for you, my hippy chick, is the wrap dress. Since the sexy 1970s, the wrap has been a godsend for modern women everywhere. The deep V-neck will lengthen your top and draw attention to your rack (always good!). Because the wrap dress is tightly belted, it will define your tiny waist. Go for stiff fabrics, such as crisp cotton, or floaty organzas and chiffon, which will skim but not cling to the hips, before flaring out.

STEP AWAY FROM THE RAIL:

- Don't bother with boring. Forget the classic black straight-cut shift dress, which will make your top seem smaller and emphasize the curve of your hips, broadening them.

- For the same reason, steer clear of any kind of all-over horizontal print or horizontal detailing, such as ruching or draping.

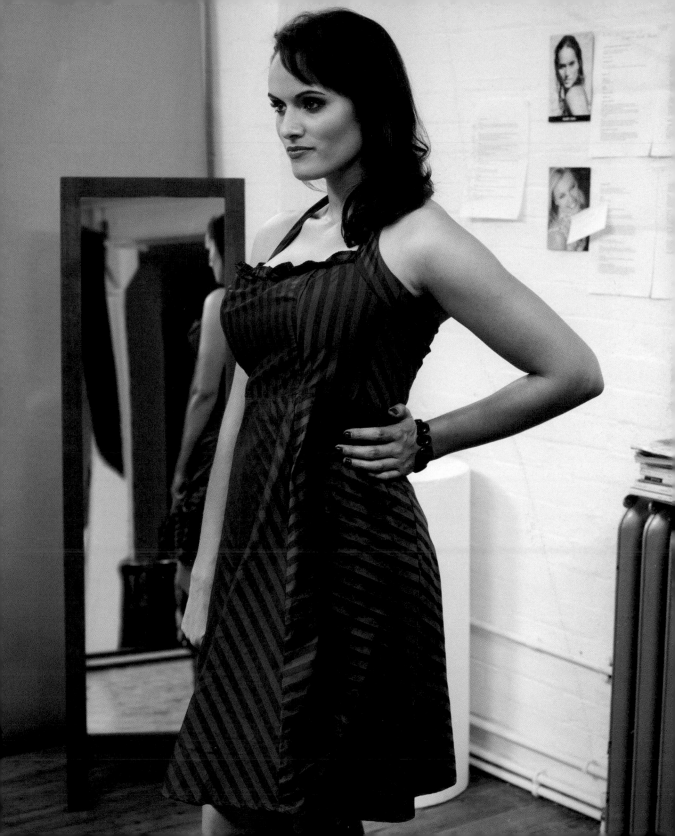

Juicy Girl's Perfect Eveningwear

Think clean lines in great colours (black tie doesn't have to be black). A strapless dress that is fitted down to your waist then skims the hips to flare out to a slightly A-line shape is perfect. Again, try stiff fabrics or floaty organza and chiffons. The A-line shape echos your shape, but the tiny top will give the illusion that you are tiny all over, and that it is just the skirt (not your hips) that are wider.

For a really jazzy event, a halter-neck plunge, floor-length gown with an A-line flared skirt would be a killer look on you!

STEP AWAY FROM THE RAIL:

- I cannot emphasize this enough: cling is so not your thing. Avoid anything bias cut or made from stretchy jersey.
- Don't even look at anything with embellishment around the middle (which will make everyone gawp at your hips).

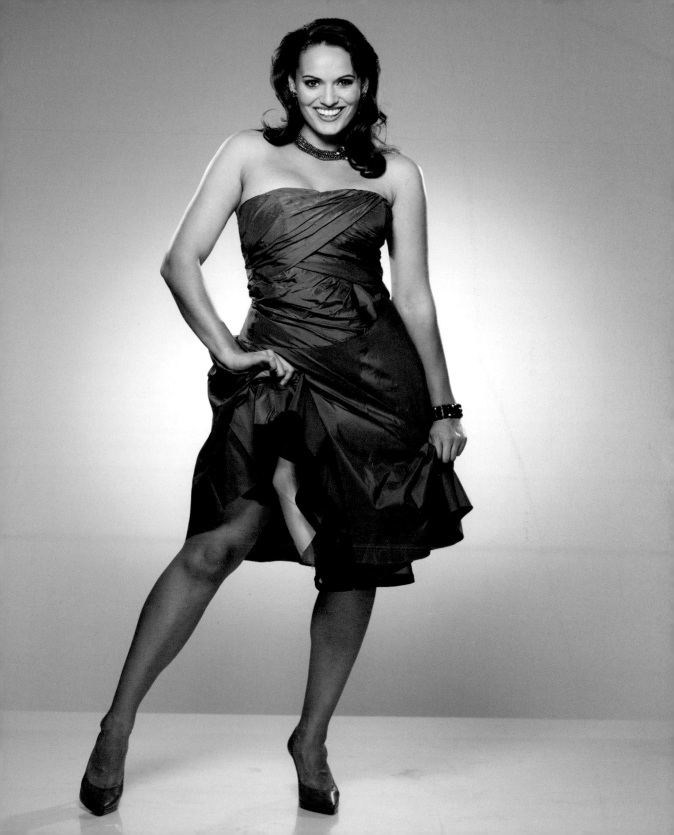

Juicy Girl's Perfect Tops

Horizontal stripes add width, so they are the perfect print for your top half. Wide-collared shirts will add breadth to your shoulders and balance the hips. Three-quarter sleeves will focus attention on your tiny waistline. Cap sleeves broaden the shoulders. Like jackets, tops should finish at the top of your hip. Thick knits will also add volume to your top half. In warmer weather, try layering thin tops.

STEP AWAY FROM THE RAIL:

- Tiny skin-tight fitted T-shirts, cropped tops and string-strap vest tops will make your top seem smaller, which will make your hips seem broader.
- A tiny buttoned-up shirt collar will over-emphasize your delicate shoulder span, as will voluminous full-length sleeves.

BEST FRIEND ADVICE: Stand up straight! (Do I sound like your mother now?) Everyone knows good posture will knock pounds off your weight, and add inches to your height (this can only be a good thing). Pear shapes in particular look bad when slouching: it emphasizes the roundness of the shoulders, and pushes the hips forward, making them seem larger.

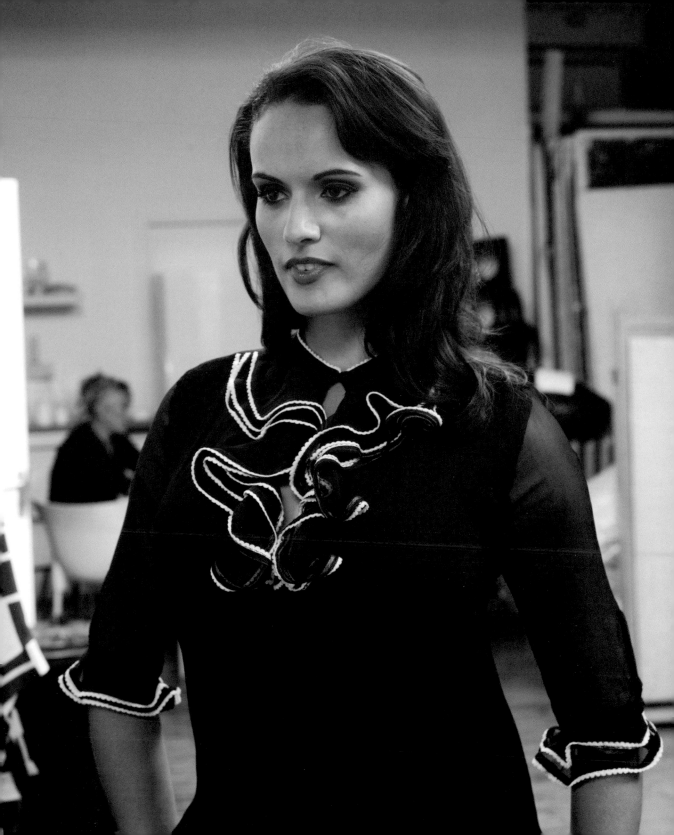

Juicy Girl's Perfect Trousers

You may have noticed that because of the width of your hips, pear-shaped ladies appear to have shorter legs. No worries: you just have to do sneaky trouser tricks to nix the hips and lengthen those legs.

Loose-leg trousers with a slightly higher waist will give you a shorter 'horizon line' (i.e. rather than wearing your waistband on the widest part of your hips). Your trousers should then skim your curves until they hit the widest part of your hips (no point adding extra volume there) then fall straight down to elongate your legs. Loose, straight ('parallel cut') trouser legs will streamline and therefore lengthen your lower body.

STEP AWAY FROM THE RAIL:

- Cropped trousers will, as the name suggests, crop your legs.
- Tight or tapered trousers will over-emphasize your bottom.
- No pleats please: they will add bulk at the waist.

BEST FRIEND ADVICE: Lady, use your noodle: don't tie a jumper around your waist to 'hide' your hips – it'll just draw more attention to the area.

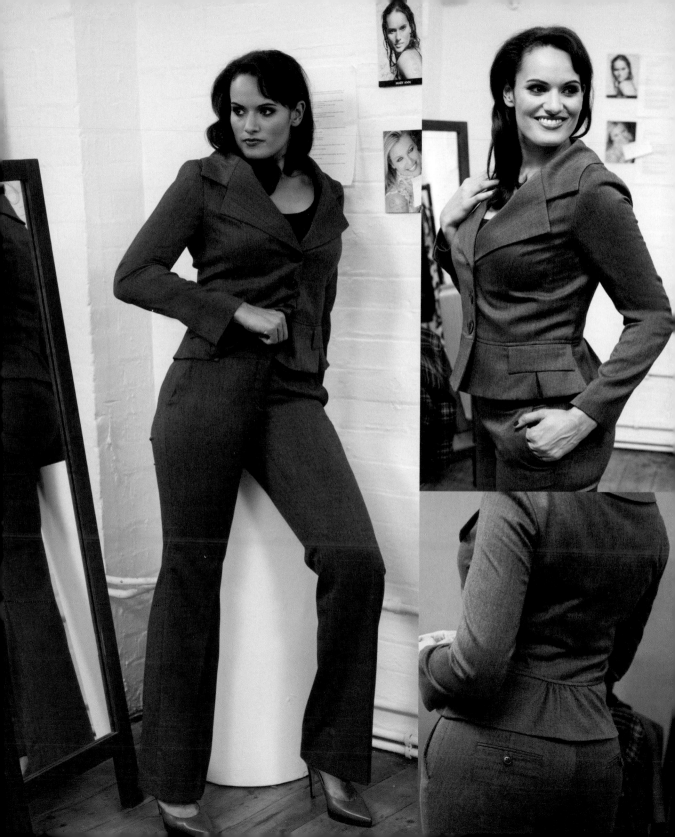

Juicy Girl's Perfect Jeans

Go boot-leg, but subtle. The best jeans to lengthen the leg will be mid-rise, in a dark wash, and straight or very slightly boot-leg with a bit of stretch. Try to find those with a wide curved waistband: jeans that are cut higher at the back will avoid any gaping at your waist. Look for big pockets in the middle of each buttock to keep everything in proportion.

Length is crucial. Jeans should hit the bottom of the ankle. But my advice is to wear them with a heel, which will help to minimize the look of wide hips even more, so the hemline can go as low as the floor when standing flat-footed.

STEP AWAY FROM THE RAIL:

- Pale jeans with horizontal shading detailing on the legs will broaden your hip area.

- Avoid small back pockets, pockets placed too far apart or no back pockets, all of which widen the area. Embroidery around the pockets will do the same thing.

Juicy Girl's Perfect Jackets

Pear-shaped ladies need shoulders that are definitely there. The structured jacket, with wider lapels and a nipped-in waist, is the best way to balance out those hips. Choose one in a stiff fabric – e.g. leather, denim or velvet – for a sharper shape. The jacket should end at the top of the hip (the narrowest bit). Having a contrasting top peeking out from underneath will add depth, making your top half seem more substantial.

STEP AWAY FROM THE RAIL:

- Loose, unstructured jackets will balance you in a bad way. You'll appear larger all over (and stuck in the 1980s).

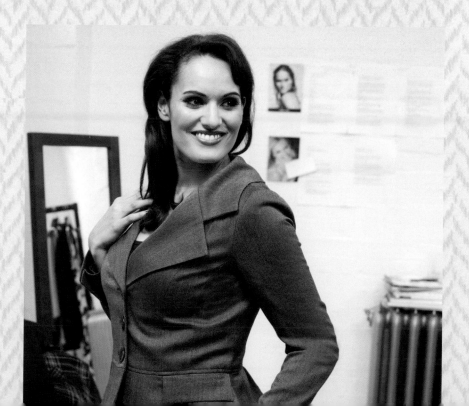

Juicy Girl's Perfect Shoes

Pointy high-heeled shoes will elongate your legs. Pointy boots look great under wide trousers.

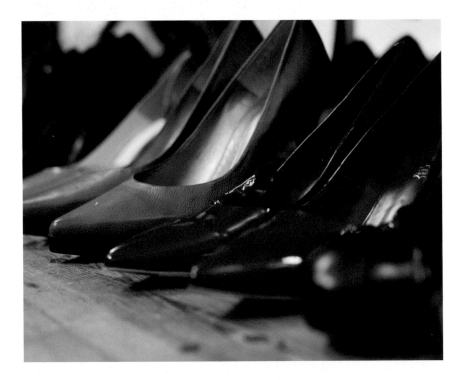

Juicy Girl's Perfect Accessories

Shoulder bags should be worn just under the arm (as opposed to being worn or carried at hip height, which will just create more width at your hips). A necklace, earrings or a brooch are great ways to highlight your gorgeous shoulders and collarbone.

SNEAKY STYLING TIP: Tie a sash belt at your waist and let the ends hang down, off to one side of your hips. This will narrow your hips, because they will appear to end where the ties are.

STEP AWAY FROM THE RACK:

- Try to avoid wearing bags slung diagonally across the body to sit at the hip, which will emphasize and broaden the area.

- A tightly belted waist may make your hips look bigger in comparison.

- Be aware that bracelets and large rings will draw attention to the hip area, and add extra bulk.

Juicy Girl's Perfect Coats

Cute on you: a three-quarter-length single-breasted coat with a slight A-line shape that flares out from the waist. Choose one with 'invisible' diagonal slit pockets, which give a false, slimmer outline to your hips. Clever, eh?

STEP AWAY FROM THE RAIL:

- Avoid boxy cut (i.e. waist-less) coats with flap pockets on the hips, which will make you appear wider.

- As a general rule, avoid garments that are fridge-shaped. Unless you want to look like a fridge!

It's not what you know, it's what you're wearing when you know it!

Juicy Girl's Rules to Remember

(Repeat after Gok, girlfriend...)

- No clingy bottoms. Go for A-line skirts and hip-skimming loose trousers.

- Avoid covering your booty with longer-line tops. All tops and jackets should end hitting the top of the hips (i.e. before the widest part).

- Keep separates lighter and more patterned on top and darker and plainer on the bottom. Darker block colours are more slimming, so use them on your lower body.

- Emphasize your boobs with a push-up bra to balance out your curves (see Underwear section).

- Don't forget: You are a beautiful English rose!

- Like any delicate fruit, you should be cared for, kept until just right for the picking and cherished for succulent, intimate enjoyment.

Booty Babe...

big butt beautiful

Count yourself lucky if you have a big, beautiful bottom. Women like Jennifer Lopez and Beyoncé have made a small fortune from having a major booty, and have made your shape the most fashionable silhouette of the moment!

And here's the science part: women store fat around the buttocks during pregnancy, so a big bouncy bottom is thought to be a sign of high fertility (frequently linked to men's subconscious attraction to women). Shake that booty, lady!

A red-hot bot is something to be proud of. Skinny chicks can now even buy padded knickers to achieve a bigger butt! Everyone wants what you've got. Sweet thought!

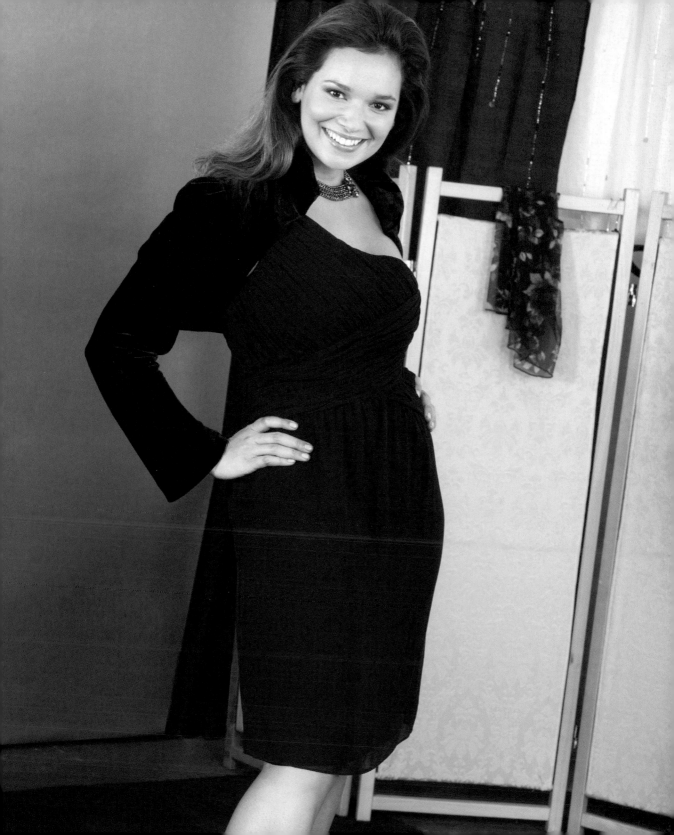

Your Magic Fashion Formula

- Show off your bottom and your waist with curve-skimming styles.
- Broaden your upper torso for balance.
- Fit-and-flare bottoms will make the most of your derrière.
- Tailor clothes to custom fit those gorgeous curves.

So tell me why, if the full, feminine bottom has so much going for it, is it the second most disliked body part for British women (after the stomach)?

Well, it has to be said that before J-Lo the bigger bottom didn't get a lot of press. Big boobs – yes; big bottoms – no. For years, Kylie's teeny hot-panted tush was being hailed as the shape to aspire to. So, perhaps not surprisingly, some bootylicious babes mistakenly thought their wonderfully raunchy rumps were simply too large. And I know this is the reason I often see gorgeous round bottoms smothered in gathered skirts, baggy trousers and jackets that cover up the curve of that perfect posterior. Criminal!

I have worked with a couple of pop stars that really have amazing, sexy, ample asses. And I'll be honest with you: when I first find out that I'm going to be styling a celebrity with a big ol' balcony butt, it is a Challenge Gok moment. Basically, I have to figure out how I'm going to work it, without constantly resorting to dresses. With this kind of depth on a derrière, magic knickers aren't exactly going to make it disappear. And why would we want it to? If anything, we need to boost those

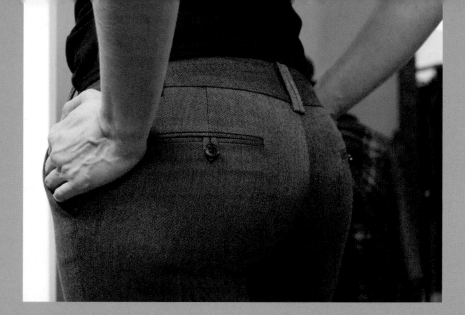

buttocks with some perk-up pants (see Underwear) to show your bottom off to its best advantage.

Also, it's worth thinking about the rest of your assets. Put it this way: if your butt is scoring twenty on the visibility scale, and your boobs are scoring five, you need to even out that ratio a bit. I'm thinking padded bra and chicken fillets (see Underwear).

Ultimately, it's all about the cut of the clothes. We really want to show off your bottom. As I mentioned in the introduction, I don't believe in figure flaws or covering up your assets. If anything, we want body-skimming clothes that will play up the size and shape of your beautiful booty. My advice: only wear tops and jackets that end below your bottom if you're worried that the sight of your gorgeous tush will make everyone else jealous.

What J-Lo and Beyoncé have in common is that they clearly love their bottoms, and this confidence comes across. When you look at them, you see women who are at ease with their bodies, rather than focusing on the clothes they are wearing. And this, my lovely, is what we're going to achieve with your wardrobe.

Booty Babe's Perfect Dresses

Your sexy silhouette is begging to be outlined in a dress. A three-quarter-sleeve square-neck tailored dress with kick pleats at the hem is your perfect check-my-curves style. The sleeves will finish at waist level, focusing attention on your slimmest part, and the square neck will broaden your shoulders, slimming your waist in comparison and balancing out your bottom. Your perfect hemline is just below knee length, to take in the full curvaceous outline of your bottom, while the kicky hem balances out the volume of your voluptuous shape.

STEP AWAY FROM THE RAIL:

- Floaty unstructured slip dresses will just hang off you, bagging at the waist and failing to show off the curve of your raunchy rump.

BEST FRIEND ADVICE: Booty beauty, your most flattering clothes will always be figure-hugging. But because of this, the fit is key. Of course, separates are your easiest option for finding the right size for your top and bottom. I know it's not exactly easy to find dresses that are perfectly shaped to your silhouette. A halter-neck wrap dress, in a not-too-clingy fabric, is a great alternative for you, because of its easy adjust-to-fit style. However, take it from me: nothing will complement your curves like a dress that really spells out your silhouette. So do consider investing in a couple of (re)tailored styles that you can always bring out to wow the crowds. (When I'm styling my bootylicious pop stars, I'm chained to that sewing machine.)

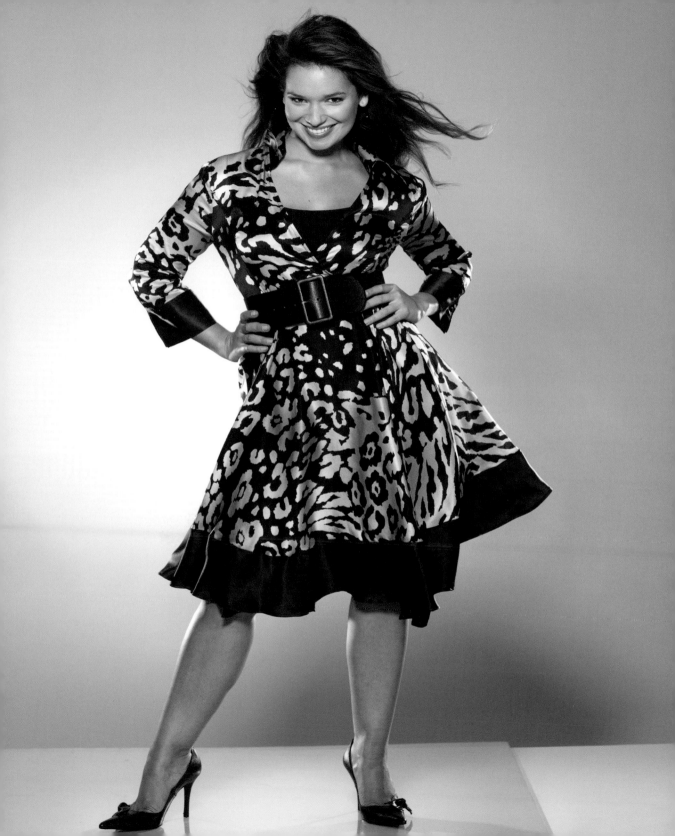

Booty Babe's Perfect Eveningwear

Foxy mama, it's all about your tiny waist for evening. Your hourglass credentials will come out in curve-skimming jersey. You can try a number of elegant necklines to broaden your upper torso: halter-neck, one shoulder, plunging, shawl collar, off-the-shoulder, or even a fitted corset top to boost your breasts. Ruching at the bust will add balance to your bottom. A sash belt will cinch in your waist.

Highlight that heiny with a fishtail skirt, train, or a waterfall ruffle coming off the bottom. Just below knee length is your perfect hemline. Consider a pretty asymmetrical hemline to break up the breadth of your lower body and show off your legs. A split will slice up your lower body, slimming and lengthening it.

A low, draped-back dress will add depth to your profile, which will balance out your pert posterior.

SNEAKY STYLING TIP: A fake-fur bolero jacket or capelet is a glamorous finishing touch to broaden your top half and balance out your bottom.

STEP AWAY FROM THE RAIL:

- Bias-cut dresses will perfectly hug your buttocks, but will also cling to your stomach and thighs and any other lumps and bumps.
- Avoid any kind of horizontal print or ruching below the waist.

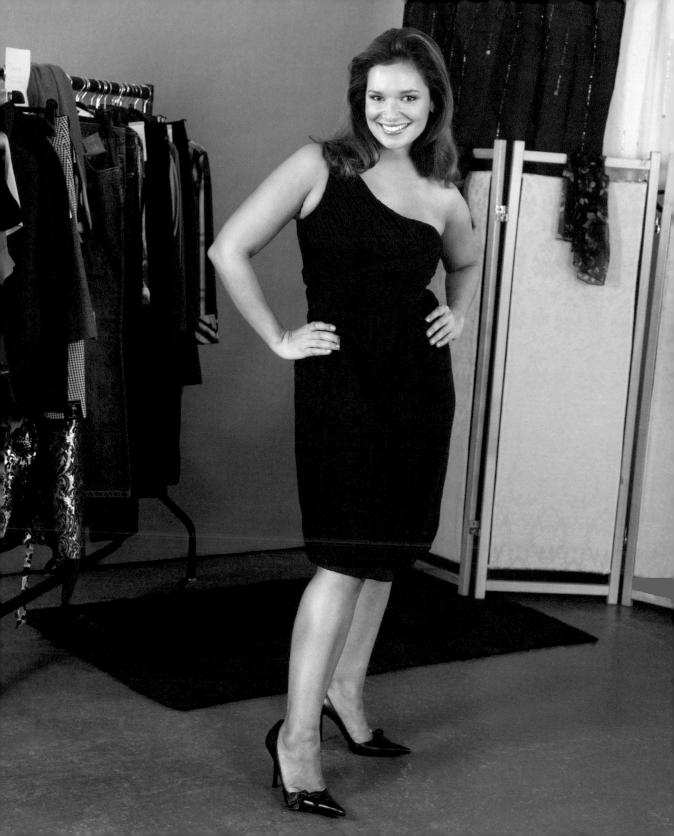

Booty Babe's Perfect Trousers

Sexy lady, I know this is your mission impossible. Your gorgeous bot will make it difficult to find trousers in a great fit, particularly at your tiny waist. Key: buy larger sizes that fit over your hips and buttocks, then take in the waist with alterations. This may seem like a big hassle, but I cannot exaggerate to you the euphoric joy of a perfect-fitting pair of trousers. For the sake of a week and twenty quid at the tailor's, you'll never regret it.

To create a longer leg line and balance your booty, choose trousers with a waistband that sits on (not below) your waist. A wide waistband will focus attention on your waist, making your bottom seem more in proportion.

Looser, straight-legged (or 'parallel cut') trousers are seriously flattering on your figure. Your trousers should skim your hips to their widest part, then fall straight down, to elongate your legs. Look for 'darts' (little vertical half-seams) above the buttocks, which will help give a form-fitting shape – you want at least two. Wearing your trousers a little longer over heels will also elongate your legs (and we love that, don't we?), making you seem slimmer all over.

STEP AWAY FROM THE RAIL:

- Don't wear colours below your waist that are lighter or brighter than those above.

- Waistband pleats will be pulled by your bottom until they balloon out, exaggerating the size of your stomach.

- Avoid narrow trouser legs, or trousers that narrow at the knees or ankles, which will make your bottom look larger in comparison.

- Also steer clear of oversized, baggy or men's trousers, which will swamp your curves. Bulky fabrics like tweed or shiny fabrics like satin, will all enlarge your lower body.

Booty Babe's Perfect Tops

Your perfect top is a colourful, long-sleeve wrap knit or shirt, ending on the jeans' waistband. The waist-cinching tie belt will highlight your tiny waist. Let the ends of the belt hang down to one side of the hips, which will visually narrow the area.

Also perfect for broadening your upper body: wide horizontal necklines (such as a square or scoop neck or a wide shirt collar) and shorter voluminous sleeves (cap sleeves, floaty sleeves, puff sleeves). Choose three-quarter-length sleeves that end at your waist, which will focus all attention there. Prints are great for emphasizing the upper body, particularly a wide horizontal stripe. A tight bright polo-neck is a foxy option to draw all eyes to your tush.

STEP AWAY FROM THE RAIL:

- Crop tops will make the two halves of your body look totally disproportionate.
- Any top that doesn't accentuate your waist will make you look huge, especially loose tops with elasticated hems.

Booty Babe's Perfect Skirts

This is your dream garment for showing off your tush. However, to make the most of your delicious derrière, we need to decrease bulk in the booty, hip and thigh area. A tulip-shape pencil skirt, fitted to your bum, and then flaring out again at the hem, couldn't be more perfect. Or try a knitted below-the-knee skirt with built-in vertical chevrons.

STEP AWAY FROM THE RAIL:

- Trust me on this: even if you love your thighs, short skirts on a bigger booty are a bad idea. Longer, on-the-knee-length hems are far better for showing off the curve of your rear, and a more sensual way to highlight your best asset.

- A-line skirts will flare out at the back ... and keep going, adding bulk without definition.

- Resist wearing a skirt that is half a size too small (but that's obvious, no?). Your skirts should be fitted, not clingy.

A day without style is like a Christmas without presents!

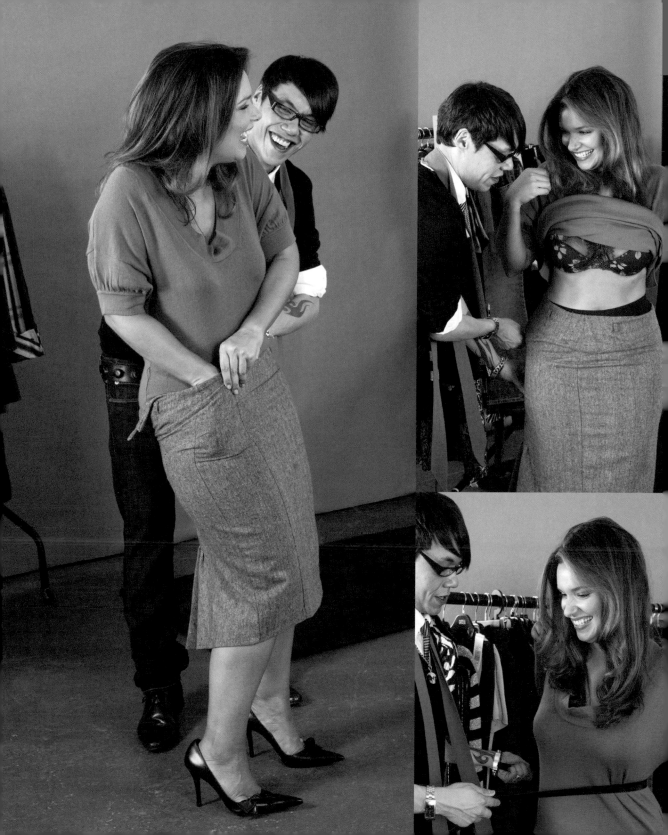

Booty Babe's Perfect Jackets

Don't be tempted to cover up your bottom with a longer-line jacket. Not only will this widen your silhouette, it will also shorten your legs. Show off that teeny waist and your beautiful booty with a shorter, waist-nipping jacket that ends at the hipbone, grazing the top of your tush.

Big lapels will give the illusion of bigger breasts, which alongside structured shoulders will help balance out your hips. But your jacket is all about the waistband: make it a big feature. You are looking for a wide, fitted waistband (or seamed waistband detailing) to focus eyes on your slimmest part. Your jacket should button from just beneath the chest, to give a fitted shape around the narrow ribcage and the illusion of a higher waist, which will make your legs appear longer. A belted jacket will also focus attention on the waist.

STEP AWAY FROM THE RAIL:

- You need structure to your silhouette, and that means stiff fabrics: thin fabrics will just crease at the waist, so avoid these.

- Cropped puffy padded jackets will give you the double-bubble silhouette of a snowman.

- High-necked jackets will 'throttle' your neck and make you appear bulkier all over.

Booty Babe's Perfect Shoes

Pointy court shoes and high-heeled boots are elegant, confident and leg-lengthening. Steer clear of round-toed shoes as these will foreshorten your legs, and their bulbous shape will over-emphasize your curves.

Flat shoes can also make you appear squat, so always think heels – even a relatively low kitten heel will give your legs some extra oomph.

Booty Babe's Perfect Accessories

Keep all accessories up top, to balance out your booty baggage. Go for a big shoulder bag tucked under the arm, big chandelier earrings, and a brooch or necklace.

STEP AWAY FROM THE RACK:

- Tiny bags held at the hip will be dwarfed by your derrière.

- Wide, low-slung belts will broaden your hips.

- Overly cinched waist belts are also a bad idea: your booty will just look bigger in comparison.

Booty Babe's Perfect Jeans

Booty cutie, this is a great time for you to be buying jeans. In recent years, manufacturers have woken up to the allure of a cushioned tush in sexy denim. Perfect for you is the curved waistband, cut higher at the back than at the front, to accommodate a larger derrière, and which avoids any gaping at the waistband. You want a mid-rise waistband (a couple of finger widths beneath your belly button), to focus on your waistline and lengthen your legs.

A straight-cut jean will also give you a longer leg line, which is very slimming. A mid-width leg will keep in proportion with your bottom, and, you'll be surprised to find, will still give you the effect of a bit of flare at the ankle.

Look for jeans with just a hint of stretch (no more than 5 per cent elastane) to hold you, but not cling. Big pockets in the middle of each buttock will keep you in proportion, and play up your pertness.

As with trousers, the hemline should go as low as the floor when standing flat-footed, so that you can wear them with leg-lengthening high heels. A darker-wash denim will be fabulously slimming on your lower torso, as will a crease down each leg.

STEP AWAY FROM THE RAIL:

- It's everyone's favourite fallback, but forget boot-cut: it will shorten most frames.

- Now is not the time to show off your tiny knees: jeans fitted too tightly there will over-exaggerate the size of your ass in comparison.

- Low-slung jeans will make your bottom look shallower, and therefore wider, as well as making your legs look shorter.

- Jeans with tiny, or no back pockets, will make your bottom seem more expansive.

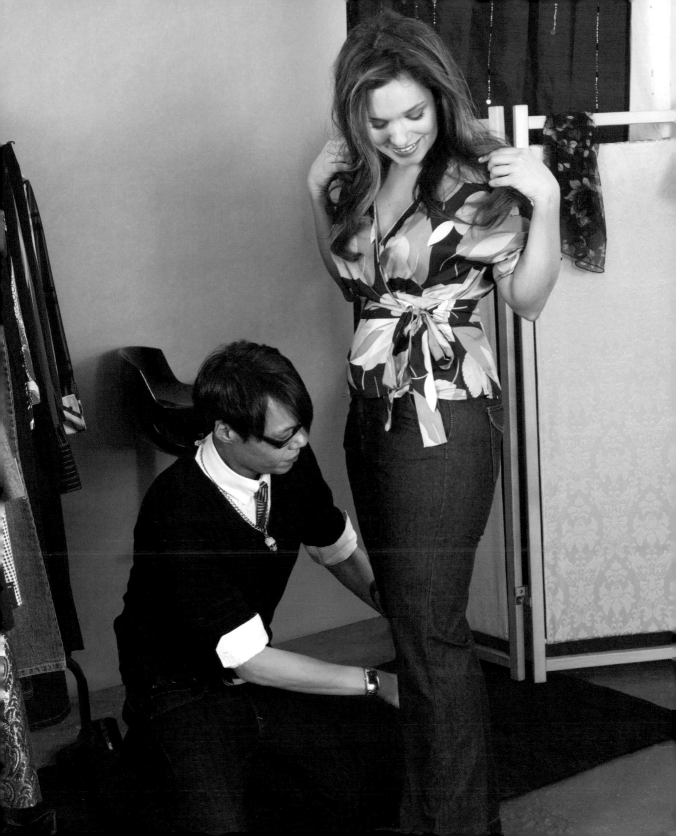

Booty Babe's Perfect Coats

In an ideal world, the weather would always be mild enough for you to wear a jacket that ends above your gorgeous peachy cheeks. Of course, when the temperature turns arctic, this is not practical.

The best style of longer coat for you is the keep-it-simple straight-cut single-breasted Crombie style, ending just below the knee. This slim column of a coat will streamline and elongate your silhouette. Again, try to find a style with some kind of focus at the waist: maybe a wide buckled belt, or a seamed waistband panel. Structured (but fitted) shoulders and wide lapels will broaden your upper torso to balance your booty. Angled hip pockets can appear to give you a slimmer silhouette. A half-belt in the small of the back can also be a great detail to subtly play up the curve of your waist and bottom.

STEP AWAY FROM THE RAIL:

- Unstructured and drop-waist styles will just broaden out your entire silhouette to match your widest part.

- Avoid gathers below the waist, which will add extra bulk.

- Steer clear of puffy padded coats, or any thick fabrics like fake fur, which will add inches to your bottom.

- Flap pockets on the hips will make that area appear wider. I always sew up my pockets.

Booty Babe's Rules to Remember

(Repeat after Gok, sweet cheeks...)

- Always ensure the curve of your waist and your bottom are defined.

- Keep skirt hems below the knee.

- Never wear loose, unstructured styles.

- Elongate your legs with wide mid-rise trousers.

- Look for jackets with a high, fitted waist.

- Remember: your beautiful booty is the look of the moment!

Petite girl...

small but perfectly formed

Gorgeous things come in small packages (and I'm not just talking about those turquoise Tiffany boxes).

Oh, to be petite but perfectly formed, just like you. When you're around, the rest of us feel like gangly, galumphing giants (thanks very much!).

Of course, you already know this, but fellas love a shorter woman (we get to feel all chivalrous). As a result, the vertically challenged lady tends to be luckier in love. A scientific journal recently proved that the majority of men favour women of below-average height (under 5'4") for long-term relationships. *Vive la différence!*

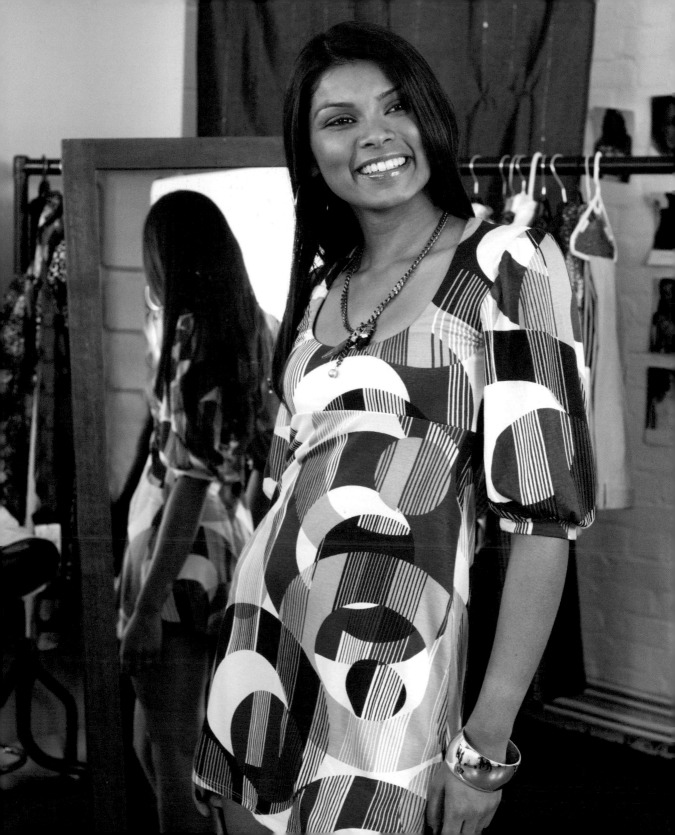

Your Magic Fashion Formula

- Keep styles simple, streamlined and straight.
- Show lots of leg.
- Skirts and dresses should end above the knee.
- Make a high-visibility statement with bright colours.

While catwalk models are all giraffes, many Hollywood actresses are tiny (partly to ensure that they don't tower over their leading men). Sarah Jessica Parker, Reese Witherspoon and Natalie Portman have all proved that there are no height restrictions when it comes to sophisticated style statements.

Fashion-wise, many high street stores are finally offering each season's key looks in scaled-down sizes, making it easier for you to avoid the traditional traps of dressing too little-girly (or, worse, too little-old-lady).

Despite being so desirable, many shorter women are frustrated by their frame, and feel overshadowed by taller friends. So, in this chapter I'm going to show you how you can hold your head high in the style stakes. And, not surprisingly, the No. 1 rule for petite chic is less is more: less width, less fuss, less clutter. But never less than fabulous.

Petite Girl's Perfect Trousers

Your trouser heroine is Audrey Hepburn. Think flat-front, lean-legged, tailored trousers. Now let's lengthen those legs of yours (sounds painful, no?): wear your hemline low (to the bottom of your high heels), and your waistband slightly higher (just under the belly button). Soft, draping fabrics, such as fine wool, will work best to create a long, fluid line.

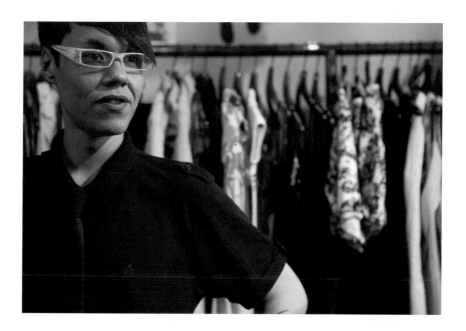

STEP AWAY FROM THE RAIL:

- Avoid pleats, pockets, baggy or low-slung combat or tracksuit trousers, which will all add the dreaded width. Even for the gym. Turn-ups will chop off your legs.

Petite Girl's Perfect Dresses

Girrrrl, let's get dressy! Dresses are the most flattering choice for you, because wearing just one colour from shoulders to knees will streamline you, making you appear taller.

Up to your neck in a garment is so not a good look for you: high necklines can make you appear squat. A low neckline slices into your torso, narrowing and elongating you.

Warning: Width is your worst enemy! The wider the style, the shorter you will appear. So, the straighter the shape, the better. A body-skimming dress will slim and lengthen your frame. Simple straight styles will also be easier to shorten if you need to make alterations (find a local tailor you can trust). And let's see those legs! Take that hemline as high as you dare.

SNEAKY STYLING TIP: Forget your torso, and focus on your legs. The longer they look, the taller you will appear as a whole. For this reason, the empire-line cut (with a horizontal seam under your bust) is perfect for you: minimum body = maximum legs!

STEP AWAY FROM THE RAIL:

- Remember: Less is more. Too many different elements to an oufit – blocks of colour, or contrasting belts or collars – will appear to chop you in half, visually shortening your body, so give them a miss.

- Big prints will overwhelm you (go for tiny prints or choose a bright colour for boldness).

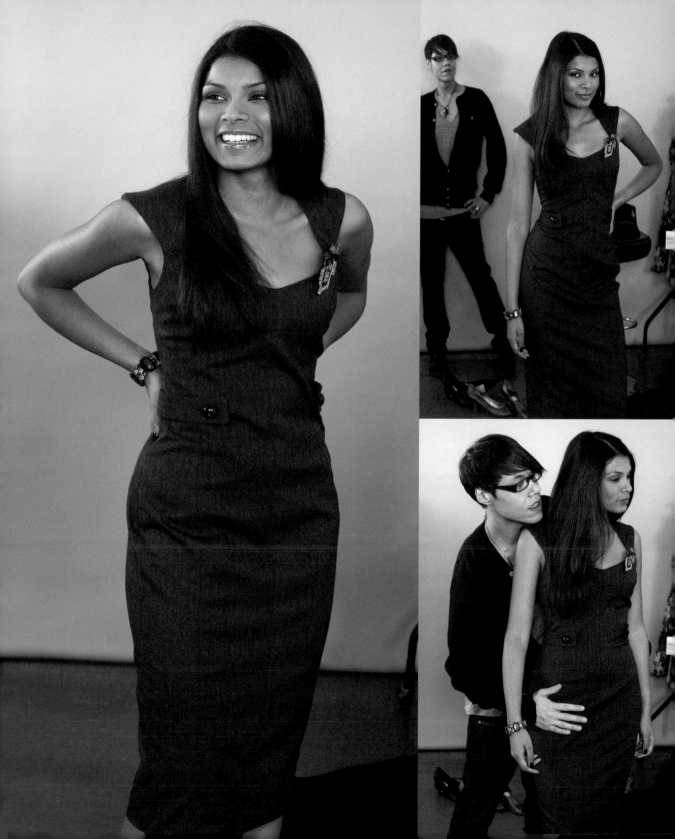

Petite Girl's Perfect Eveningwear

Guess what, doll? The 'straight, slim and simple' story is the same for eveningwear. Halter-neck, strapless, one shoulder or strappy styles are all great looks for you. A hem that is shorter at the front than at the back will lengthen and showcase legs, and again, keep it above the knee. A split can be foxy on a straight dress.

Narrow vertical pleating or seaming will draw the eye down and elongate you. The dress code might be black tie, but when it comes to colour choose anything but black. For maximum physical presence go for eye-catching colours, bold and bright. Light-reflecting shiny fabrics like satin will also give you high visibility. Own your space!

STEP AWAY FROM THE RAIL:

- Avoid anything too fussy: bows, ruffles, puff sleeves, etc. will be too little-girly, as well as make you look wider and shorter.
- Avoid dresses with two-tone blocks of colour that appear to be separates.
- Steer clear of drop-waisted styles, which will reverse the opposite of your longer legs/shorter torso fashion formula.

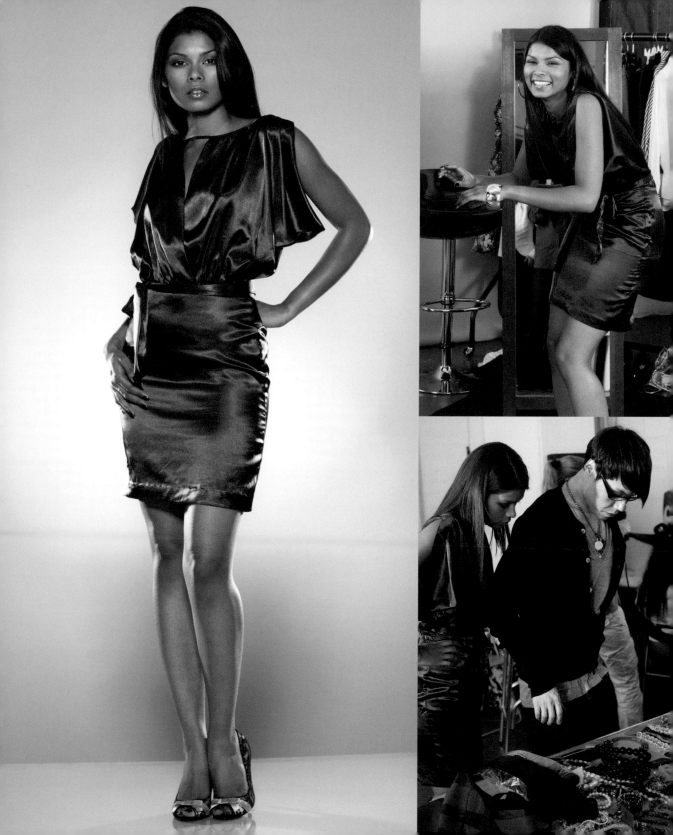

Petite Girl's Perfect Tops

Keep tops simple. As ever, too many things going on in an outfit will chop you up. A slim-fit one-colour V-neck knit will streamline your upper body. And don't be afraid to be sexy: show off a little décolletage – the vertical slice will also elongate your shape.

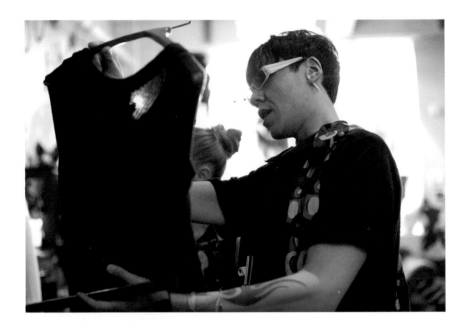

STEP AWAY FROM THE RAIL:
- Avoid sloppy oversized sweatshirts, shirts and jumpers, and excessive layering. Crop tops will do just that.

Petite Girl's Perfect Shoes

A closed, pointy-toe shoe, cut away at the arch of the foot for maximum leg exposure, will lengthen your lower body.

Better yet, for real streamlining choose a shoe colour that tones with your bare legs, or a shoe with invisible straps, or match the colour of your tights to your shoes to visually lengthen the legs.

A mid-height kitten heel will keep you in proportion. But don't be afraid of flats: round-toed ballet pumps can look very chic on petite women.

STEP AWAY FROM THE RACK:

- Avoid extra-pointed shoes, which may seem too long for your height.

- Also steer clear of boots (I know: heartbreaker!). These are a bad idea because they will crop the length of your legs. Ditto ankle straps.

BEST FRIEND ADVICE: I often see petite women teetering around in stilt-like clumpy high heels like wedges or platforms. You know what? You're not fooling anyone, and this actually just draws everyone's attention to your lack of height. You are better off keeping your heels in proportion to your foxy frame, and getting noticed for all the right reasons instead.

Petite Girl's Perfect Skirts

A slim-line pencil skirt looks cool and classy and is endlessly versatile: tweed in the office; denim at the weekend; slinky silk on hot dates. See what I mean? Best worn to just above the knee, and tapered in at the hemline to add sexy curves to your hips. Once found in the perfect cut, buy in every colour!

STEP AWAY FROM THE RAIL:

- An A-line or 1950s-style gathered skirt will make you look wider (and just a little too Tinkerbell).

- Hems with a band of ruffle or contrasting colour will cut you in two and shorten the leg area.

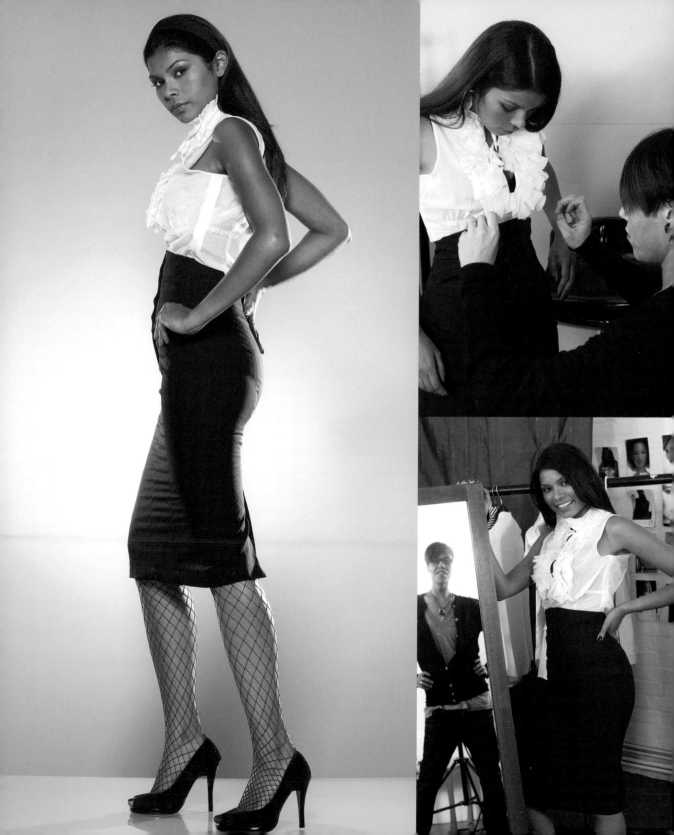

Petite Girl's Perfect Jackets

Another key piece for your wardrobe, nearly as important as the dress, is the structured short jacket. Tailoring adds an important element of take-me-seriously sophistication to your look. You want a shapely nipped-in waist (on you and the jacket). Look for a waistline that is slightly higher than your natural one (the jacket equivalent of the empire line). The hem should sit on top of the hip. Look for slimmer sleeves to keep bulk and width to a minimum on top. Narrow vertical pinstripes are a great print to stretch you out, and also majorly flattering for trousers and skirts.

STEP AWAY FROM THE RAIL:

- Boxy or bulky jackets or double-breasted styles will broaden and therefore shorten you.

- A puffa jacket would be silhouette suicide.

When you look like a million dollars, everything is possible.

Petite Girl's Perfect Accessories

For your accessories it's all about proportion and polish. Keep bags small and worn close to the body. Jewellery should be delicate; belts and watch straps narrow. Choose sophisticated accessories that command respect, in deluxe leather and suede, and in confident original colours such as purple or olive.

Length lengthens: so choose a narrow scarf looped around the neck with the two ends hanging down, or a long, fine necklace to draw the eye down and slim the body. Ultimately, always try to keep accessories to a minimum for a more streamlined appearance. Like I said, less is more. Except when it comes to shopping...

STEP AWAY FROM THE RACK:

- Long, strapped or outsized bags, giant beads, big bangles and wide belts will all swamp you.

Petite Girl's Perfect Jeans

Girlfriend, everyone is going to tell you that if you're petite the best style of jeans for you are boot-cut. Except me. Remember that width thing we were talking about? That's why you don't want flared hems on your jeans. The best way to lengthen your body is with darker wash straight-cut jeans with a crease to elongate and slim the leg. Focus first on a cut that fits in the waist, hip and bottom. Then get them shortened; but again, wear them extra, extra long (hem to the bottom of your favourite high heels) for extra inches of leg.

SNEAKY STYLING TIP: Wearing your top tucked in, or hitting your waist-band, will make legs look longer.

> STEP AWAY FROM THE RAIL:
>
> - Like boot-cut styles, fussy fading and decorative detailing like beading and embroidery will only shorten the leg (and make you look like a trend-obsessed teenager).
> - Keep your jeans belt-free to avoid breaking up the line of your legs.

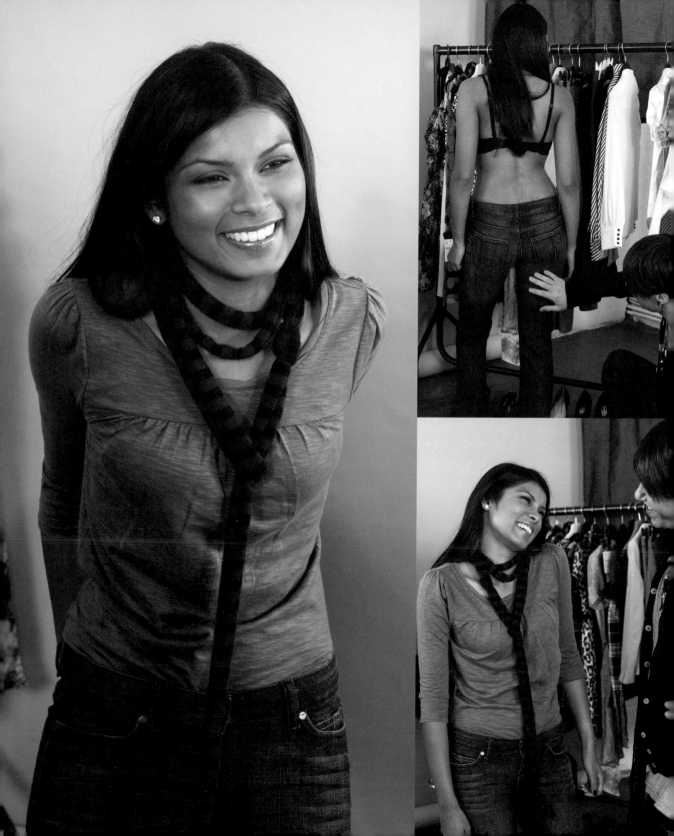

Petite Girl's Perfect Coats

Your coats should be grown-up, not girly. This means the simple sophistication of a single-breasted, slim and straight Crombie-style coat. One long knee-length column will stretch that silhouette. And don't automatically buy black! Choose your outerwear in more attention-seeking shades so that you can always arrive (and exit) in style.

STEP AWAY FROM THE RAIL:

- Any loose coat, from a baggy trench to an edge-to-edge coat, will make you shrink by inches.
- Long coats or funnel necks will swamp you.
- Steer clear of rounded collars and big buttons, which will look way too cutesy and kiddie on you.

Choose your wardrobe like you choose your lovers – effortless, timeless and good on the bedroom floor!

Petite Girl's Rules to Remember

(Repeat after Gok, gorgeous girl…)

- Necklines low, hemlines high.

- Accessories should be polished and in proportion to your frame.

- Keep all eyes on you in bold, bright colours.

- Elongate your silhouette: slim and vertical, not wide and horizontal.

- Remember: shorter torso, longer legs, taller lady.

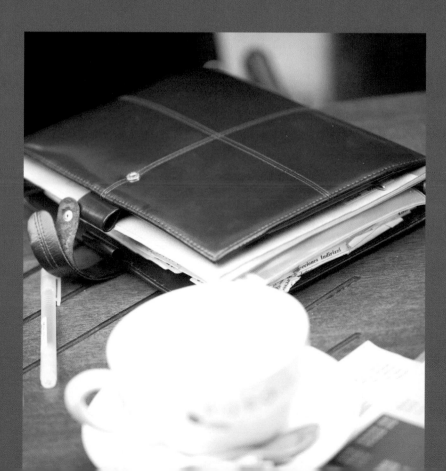

Sexy Broad...

no curves but who cares

Honey, you're a real broad. Your broad body and straight up-and-down figure give you a body type known in fashion as the Apple. And that's exactly what you are: sexy, fruity and juicy.

It's fun to create curves: a sexy flare here, a ruched detail there, some gorgeous colours and eye-foxing prints.

You're as curvaceous and feminine as an hour-glass silhouette, just in a more rounded way...

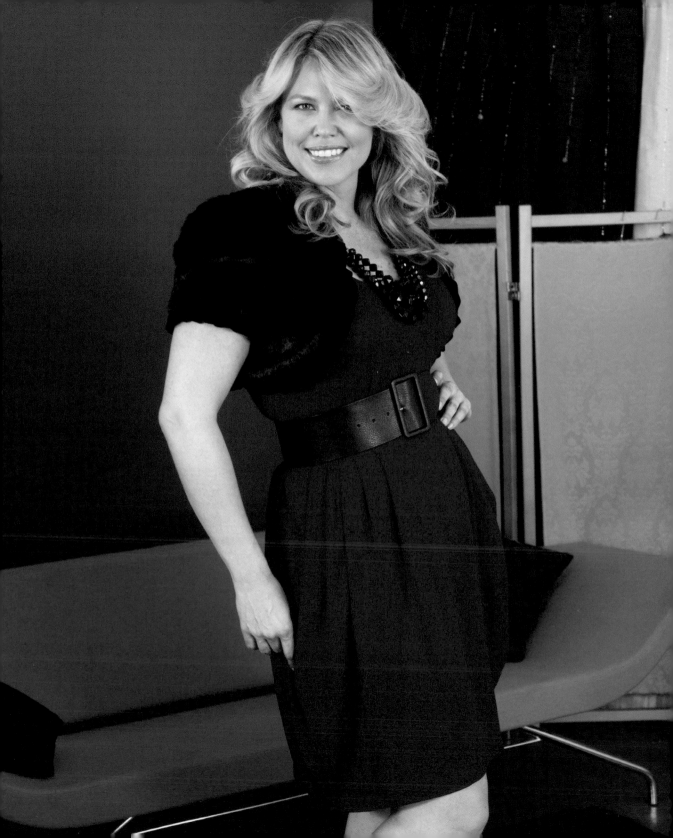

Your Magic Fashion Formula

- Add shape and volume to your upper and lower torso.
- Raise waistbands to emphasize your waist.

Of course, you probably crave a figure of eight (instead of a 0), because what you want most in the world is some kind of waist. Well, you're not the only one. In 1951, the average British woman had a 27.5-inch waist. Now, the average woman's waist measures 34 inches (that's a growth of more than an inch a decade!).

I often see waistless women trying to conceal their lack of curves in baggy, shapeless clothes. Big mistake. Shapeless clothing will always make you look wider. Instead, we need to focus on your best assets with shapely, structured clothing.

Obviously, the belt is your best friend. Before waist belts became a major fashion statement, I used to buy those wide elasticated nurses' belts to use on shoots. I've laced lots of sexy broads into corsets (it certainly works for pop stars, but obviously that look is a little high-maintenance for everyday life).

Most of all, it's important for you not to blow your waistlessness out of proportion. You only need the slightest hint of an indentation to give the impression of a waist. If a thick waist is your main problem, that's not so bad. It's a really easy one to solve, once you know some sneaky styling tricks.

I think you'll be amazed by the curves we can achieve, with just clever dressing. And don't worry, there won't be any need to wrestle you into a corset (unless, of course, you want me to!).

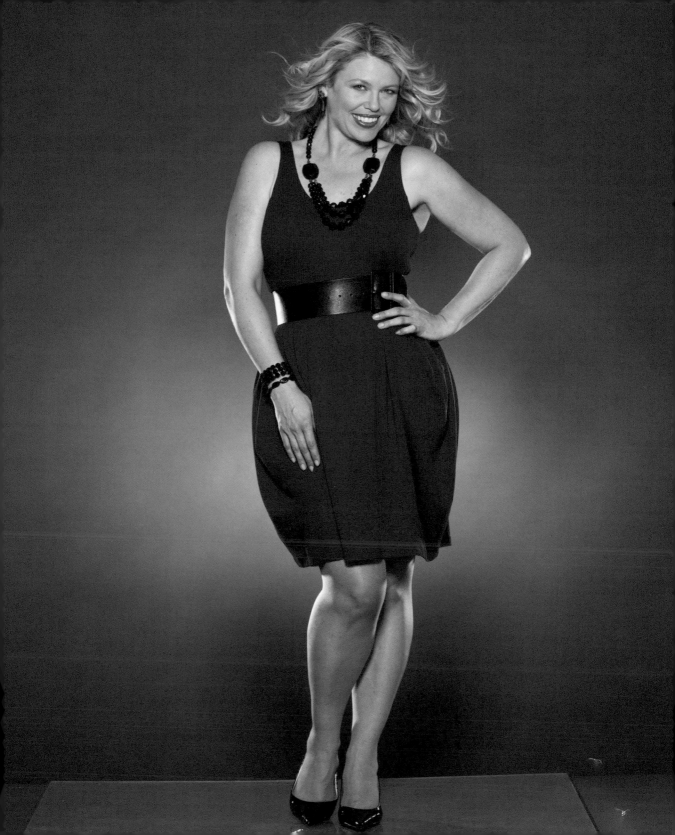

Sexy Broad's Perfect Dresses

What a waist! That's what we want everyone to say when they see your figure. And you know how we're going to do that? We're going to show off your ribcage (always the skinniest part of the body) and pretend it's your waist! Naughty.

Empire-line styles create a high waistline just under the bust, making the body beneath look much longer, and therefore slimmer. Emphasizing the bustline with a ribbon tie, or some other detailing, will also help to draw the eye upwards, and away from your midsection.

A great style of day dress for you will be a waist-wasping wraparound dress with a deep V-neck. The vertical neckline will slice into your torso, breaking up your broad body.

Another smart trick: volume on the sleeves and skirt will make your midsection seem slimmer in between.

On all dresses, printed fabrics are a great idea for creating interest and distracting from a straight silhouette, which will only be starkly outlined by solid, plain colours.

SNEAKY STYLING TIP: Layering is a great way to add depth and interest to an outfit and distract from a solid torso. Try layering a contrasting camisole top under a dress to give a pop of colour, or adding a striking belt at your waist.

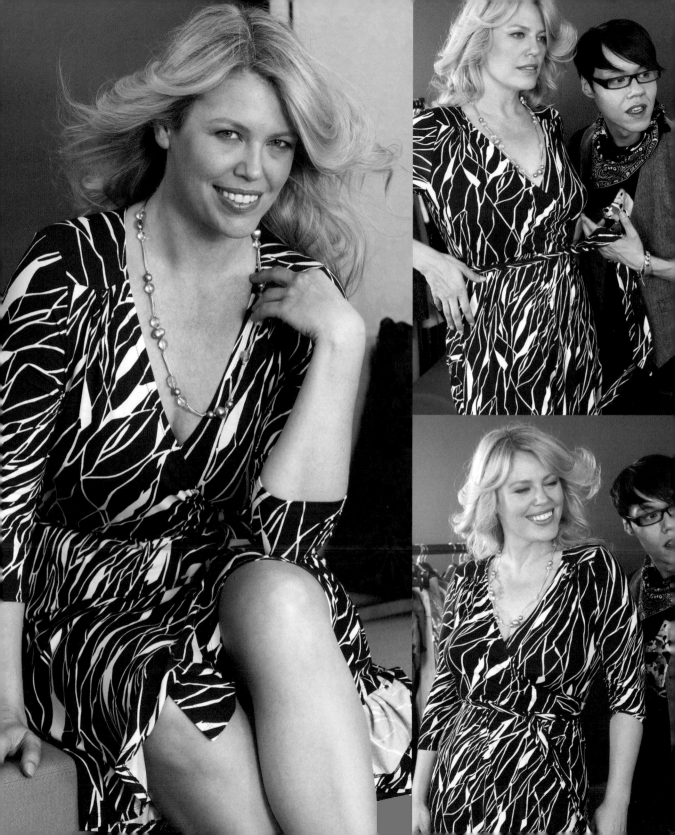

Sexy Broad's Perfect Eveningwear

For those with broad shoulders, a strapless prom dress with an A-line skirt is a great way to slim the torso and add angles at your midsection, creating hips and a waist. Alternatively, a deep V halter-neck empire-line dress, with high ruched waistband, will make a thick waist appear thinner.

STEP AWAY FROM THE RAIL:

- Avoid straight up-and-down shift dresses, drop-waisted dresses, and tenty empire-line dresses that fall softly from the bustline: all these will cover your lack of curves, but they won't give you a waist.

- Clingy, straight styles will just make your midsection the focus.

Always dress to be undressed.

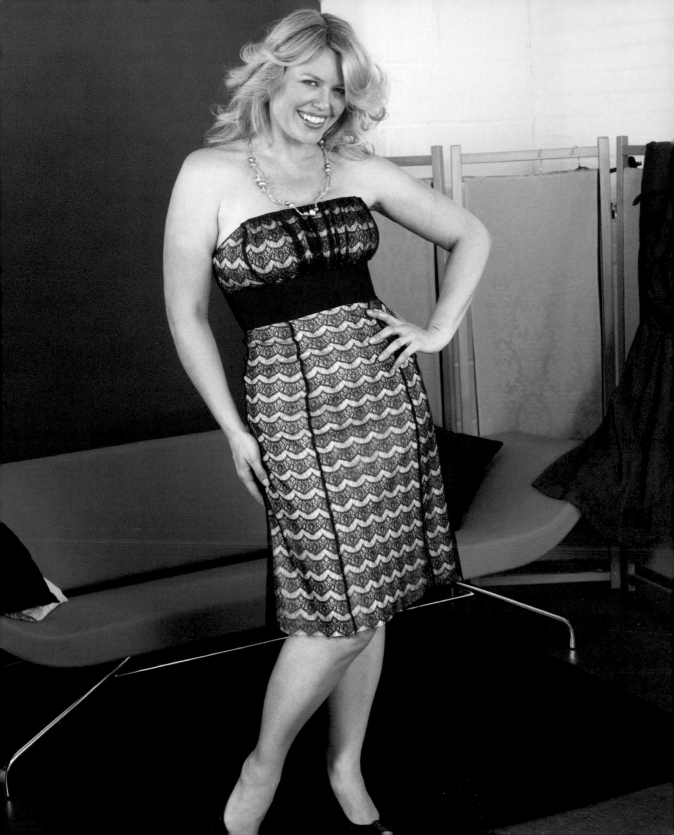

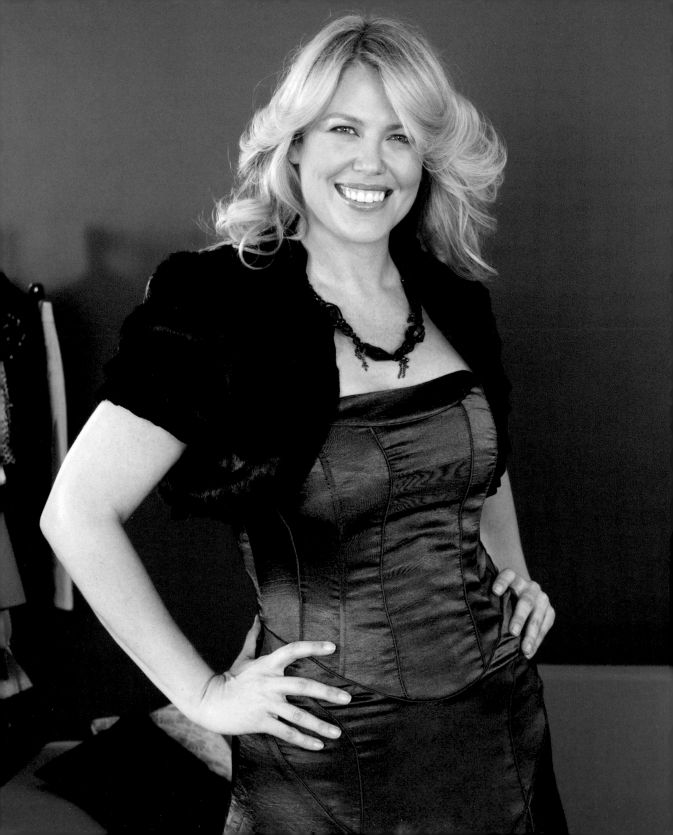

Sexy Broad's Perfect Trousers

From the waist down, it's important for you to add a little volume, to make your midsection seem narrower in comparison. So for trousers, a flowy style with wide, straight legs will give you a smaller waist.

A mid-rise waistband will keep your legs looking as long as possible (helping your figure to look longer and more vertical, and less wide and horizontal). A curved waistband is also a good trick: it'll give the suggestion of shapely curves to your silhouette too.

A crease down the front of your trousers will vertically bisect the legs, making them appear slimmer, and the continuous line will further elongate the lower body. In fact, to balance the wider cut, you should wear your trousers slightly too long, with pointy high heels to lengthen and slim those legs.

STEP AWAY FROM THE RAIL:

- Pleated trousers will add bulk to your middle, as will an elasticated waistband.
- Avoid turn-ups, which will make your legs appear shorter.

BEST FRIEND ADVICE: Posture is very important for you. It's easy to create curves with a sexy hands-on-hips posing. And ensuring one leg is always ever-so-slightly further forward will add angles to your midsection.

Sexy Broad's Perfect Skirts

A skirt is the perfect opportunity for you to soften your silhouette. Again, you're looking to create subtle volume from the waist down. An A-line or softly flared style will create hips, and therefore a waist.

With a broad body, you need a long enough skirt to balance it out, so that the slimming vertical line has more impact than the horizontal width. A hemline finishing just below knee-length will create the perfect balance. Curved waistbands will appear to narrow the waist. Asymmetric hemlines will de-emphasize the width of the body and give shape to the hips.

Use prints and contrasting colours and layers of clothing to create shape. Attention-seeking patterns, and embellishment such as sequins or embroidery, will add interest to the lower body, drawing the eye, and making this area seem larger than the midsection.

STEP AWAY FROM THE RAIL:

- Forget styles with gathers or pleats on the waist; all volume should be below or above the waistline, not on it.
- Straight pencil skirts will make your torso a shapeless block.

Sexy Broad's Perfect Jackets

If you have a straight torso, the best way to create an instant hourglass silhouette is with a curvy-cut single-breasted jacket.

Structured shoulders will make the waist appear narrower in comparison, as well as subtly lengthening (and therefore slimming) the upper body.

Your jackets should button just under the chest, to give a higher 'waist' line on your slim ribcage, which will streamline your midsection.

The jacket should finish just below the hipbone to accentuate the fitted waist. Angled hip pockets and a gently flaring peplum hemline will help create shapely hips and the suggestion of a slimmer waist. And don't forget, you can always buckle a contrasting belt over your jacket, *très* hot!

Narrow sleeves will reduce an overall impression of bulk on the torso. Or choose short-sleeved styles. Rounded lapels or any interesting lapels will accentuate the chest, and add curves.

SNEAKY STYLING TIP: Wearing fitted jackets open will reveal just a long, vertical line of clothing beneath, which slims and elongates the body.

STEP AWAY FROM THE RAIL:

- Boxy jackets with a square outline will make you look even less shapely.
- Jackets that end at the waist will make you look chunkier.
- Avoid jackets that are too small to button comfortably (a fitted jacket will give you curves, a too-tight jacket will only make you look larger).

Sexy Broad's Perfect Tops

Tops should be high-waisted, fitted, and have volume in the sleeves and flare at the hem.

Exposing a little skin at the collarbone helps shape the torso. But keep the necklines vertical (deep V and scoop necks) rather than horizontal (slash necklines and off-the-shoulder styles), finishing lower than the collarbone, to elongate and slim the upper body. Wear necklines as low as you like, and layer contrasting tops to add interest and depth to distract from the straight lines of your midsection.

Prominent collars and capped or floaty cape sleeves will also broaden and soften the shoulders, making the waist slimmer in comparison.

Styles should skim the ribcage from the bustline down: the best top for this is a V-neck wrap top, which is adjustable so it can be fitted to the body. A fitted shirt is also a good style for you: think of it as a lightweight version of the figure-fixing jacket.

Any detailing around the waist is a great idea: from decorative stitching or seaming, to draped or ruched fabric or a contrasting sash, bow or belt. Just make sure the end result is still fitted to the waist.

All tops should hit the hipbone. A little flare at the hem will help give the illusion of hips. Also, look for tops that have small side slits to give a bit of a kick at the hem.

SNEAKY STYLING TIP: Try a form-fitting waistcoat with a tightly cinched back-strap (this is another of my favourite waist-creating tricks on shoots) to leave a slimming central panel of clothing beneath.

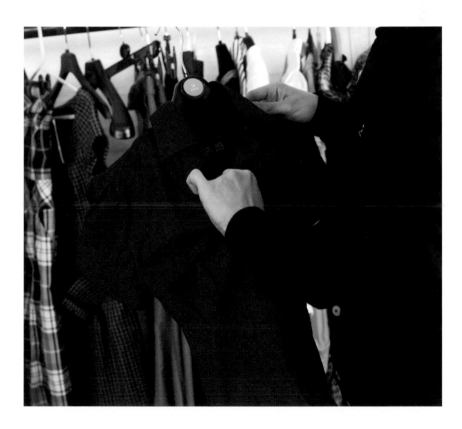

Sexy Broad's Perfect Shoes

Again, brightly coloured shoes will add interest to your outfit. A long pointed-toe shoe will balance the width of your body. High heels are essential for lengthening your legs. Low-cut shoes (at the toes and foot arch) will also add much-needed inches to your legs.

STEP AWAY FROM THE RACK:

- Rounded toes may disappear under wider trousers.

- Flat shoes won't help with lengthening those legs (try a small kitten heel instead).

- Ankle straps will add curves to the calves, but will also break up the line of the leg, shortening your lower body.

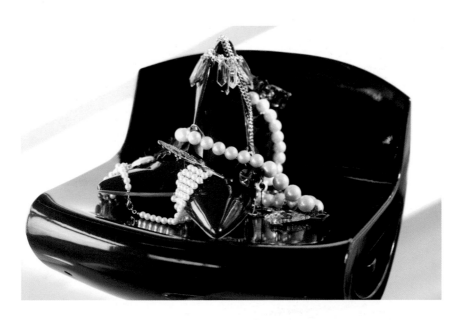

Sexy Broad's Perfect Accessories

Of course, the belt is going to be your perfect accessory. Whether it's a wide waist belt, a sexy corset-style belt, a sash, a ribbon tied in a bow or a wide belt worn on the hips to make the waist seem slimmer in comparison, you can never have too many.

Belts that are asymmetrical, curved or shaped or multicoloured will be particularly flattering (shaping your midsection like a curved waistband). Tie belts at the waist and leave the ends to hang down to one side of the body, visually narrowing that area.

Also, try adding bright punches of colour with shoes, belts and bags in contrasting colours. This will add interest and depth to your outfit, breaking up the width of your silhouette. Bags are a great way to add crazy prints to an outfit, for the styling-shy.

A long, narrow scarf looped around the neck with the ends hanging down the body will elongate your torso.

STEP AWAY FROM THE RACK:

- Narrow belts emphasize the broadness of your body or just get 'lost' in your mid-section.

- Avoid bags that hang at waist height; this will just accentuate the width of your midsection.

- A tiny bag may also make your body seem broader in comparison.

Sexy Broad's Perfect Jeans

You're looking for jeans that are the same shape as your perfect trousers. It's easy to find styles that have a wide curved waistband in jeans (these have been designed for women with an ample booty, but will work brilliantly for you to give the impression of curvaceousness at your waist). So look for a mid-width, mid-rise jean. A dark wash will be more flattering and slimming on your legs.

High-set back pockets will add shape to the bottom, and lengthen legs.

STEP AWAY FROM THE RAIL:

- A low-slung waistband would be a mistake, because it will just make your legs look shorter, and your torso longer, which puts all the focus on your midsection.
- You want mid-width straight legs, not baggy jeans.
- Front pockets will emphasise your midriff, as will any 'whiskering' shading in that area. Even if you have slim legs, avoid skinny styles, which will just make your torso seem wider in comparison.

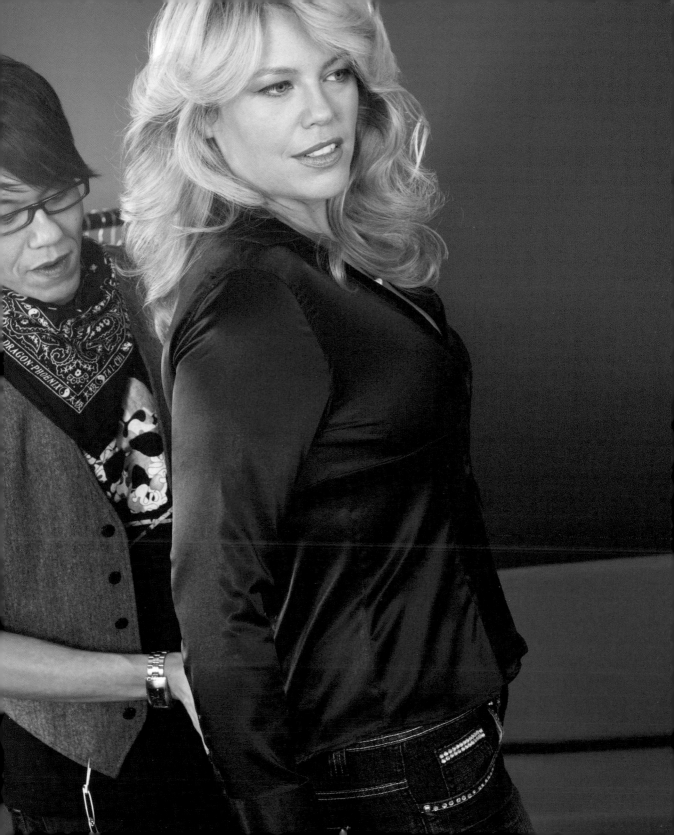

Sexy Broad's Perfect Coats

A straight, single-breasted style finishing at the knee will create one long column to elongate and slim your silhouette, making you seem taller and leaner. An open neckline will focus on your slimmest parts: your collarbone and slim neck.

High waistband detailing will lengthen and de-emphasize the waist. Hip pockets will add interest and shape, and make the waist seem slimmer in comparison.

This is the one garment you should buy in a plain colour (you're going for a lengthening, streamlining effect here, like with your trousers and jeans). Even so, a coloured coat in rich tones like chocolate, purple, navy or burgundy will give a softer silhouette. A coat in a flat black will sharpen your outline, making the width of your figure even more obvious.

Again, leave your coat unbuttoned to reveal just a long, thin sliver of clothing beneath: very slimming.

STEP AWAY FROM THE RAIL:

- Avoid belts: a coat is too bulky to cinch. In particular, a fabric belt will get lost in your torso.

- Avoid thick bulky fabrics like fake fur or thick boucle wool, which will widen your silhouette.

- Double-breasted rows of buttons will draw the eye line outwards, adding breadth to your figure.

- Never choose high-collared styles that cover up your slim neck.

Sexy Broad's Rules to Remember

(Repeat after Gok, girlfriend...)

- Don't choose clothes with a straight, shapeless silhouette.

- Add interest by layering clothes, choosing printed fabrics and accessorizing like crazy.

- Keep the waistline high, worn empire-line style on the ribcage.

- Elongate the torso with open, low vertical necklines.

- Remember: it's easy to add a waist!

Admit it, you can't wait to go shopping, can you, my Fruity Apple? I can hear the wolf whistles already....

Curvy Girl...

hourglass is the new black

Lucky you, sweetie! You've got curves to die for. Was there ever a more classic symbol of sexy gorgeousness than the hourglass silhouette? You, honey, are all woman.

The average size for women in the UK is a 16, and to me there's nothing more glamorous than a size-16 woman in a corset. Hollywood's most enduring screen goddesses – Marilyn Monroe, Sophia Loren and Jayne Mansfield – all had that fabulous figure-of-eight shape.

Even before you step into your clothes, you are 1950s movie-star glamour personified.

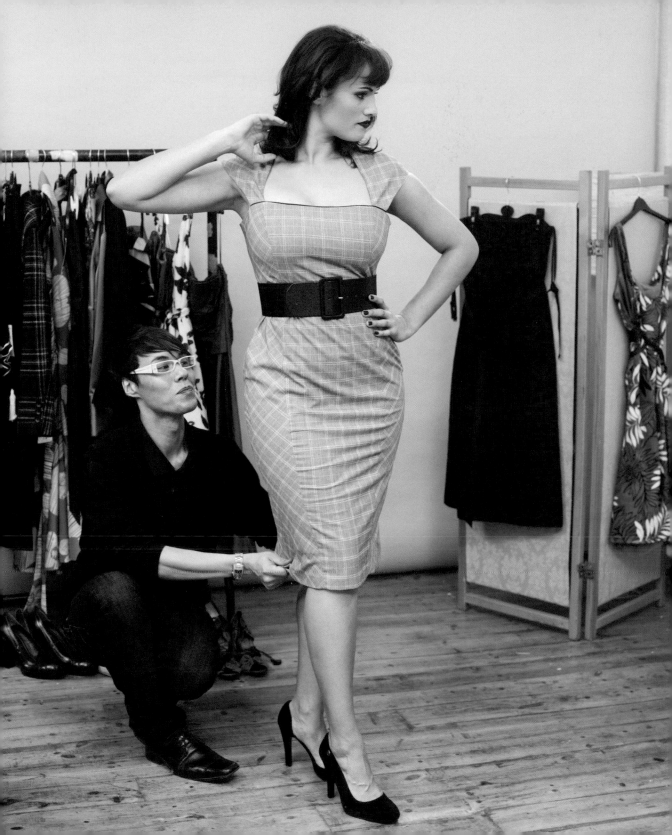

Your Magic Fashion Formula

- Boost boobs, tone tummy, skim hips and work that tiny waist.

So why do I see women who are dying to keep those killer curves under wraps, hidden beneath schlumpy tops, loose layers and baggy trousers? Madness! Often the reason is that my gorgeous hourglass girls have been looking at those skinny models in magazines and thinking, 'I'm not like that.'

Maybe you're not. But even today, the perfect proportions of the hourglass figure are still very much a modern (male) obsession: from Scarlett Johansson (dubbed The New Marilyn) and Salma Hayek to Catherine Zeta-Jones and sexy domestic goddess Nigella Lawson.

The beauty of an hourglass figure is in its symmetry and perfect proportions. Covering up your curves with baggy, dowdy clothing is the worst thing you can do...other than cutting them off with cosmetic surgery. So forget loose and shapeless clothes, and instead think sensual and shapely.

It's time for a lesson in dressing. Here's the right capsule wardrobe for my curvy girls!

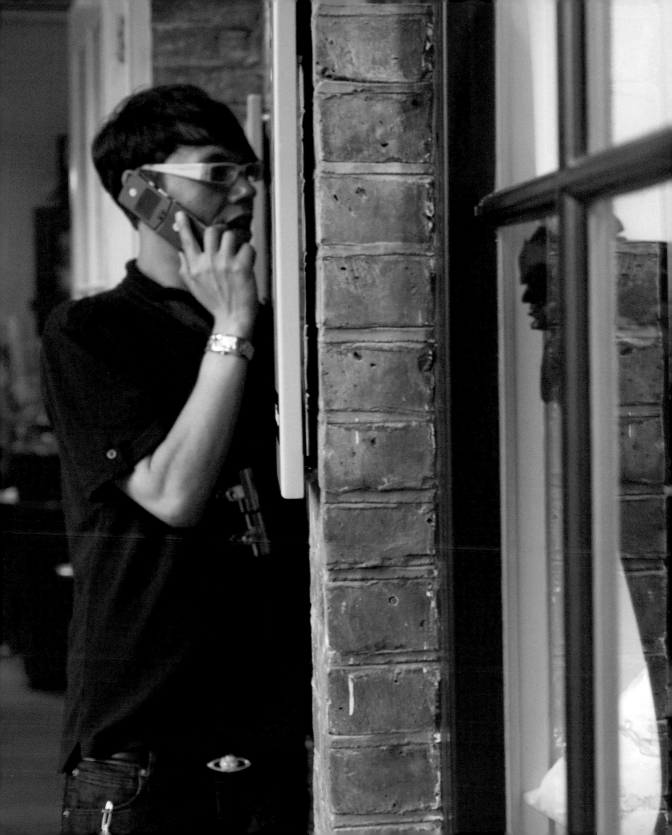

Curvy Girl's Perfect Dresses

The best dress shape for you will always be the classic 1950s frock: with a fitted top, tightly tailored waist and a wide pleated or gathered A-line shape skirt. Remember: we want to boost your boobs, tone the tummy, skim those hips and work that tiny waist.

Low, open necklines will always be best for you. Show off that beautiful collarbone with a sweetheart or scoop neckline.

Strapless styles look wonderful as a summer sundress in printed cotton. Add a knitted shrug if you are arm-shy.

A dress with a belt at the waist will cinch you in, corset-style. Basically, this is a dress with a Wow waist, and you're a girl with a Wow waist, so it's a match made in heaven!

For eveningwear, the 1950s frock will also go down a storm. In darker colours it's *très* sophisticated. Think Parisian chic, epitomized by Christian Dior and Chanel. A deep V neck will work wonders on your boobs, and all the men you meet! A wide contrasting ribbon tied around your waist in a bow, is a simple but sophisticated touch (and a great way to add a kick of colour to slimming black). Plus, you can let the ends hang down over your stomach area if you are having one of those days when you don't want to show it off – sneaky, huh?

STEP AWAY FROM THE RAIL:

- Avoid skin-tight dresses in stretchy jersey: this will highlight any lumps and bumps, which will distract from your awesome silhouette. There's a fine line between va-va-voom and vulgar with the hourglass silhouette. Let's keep it classy, lady.

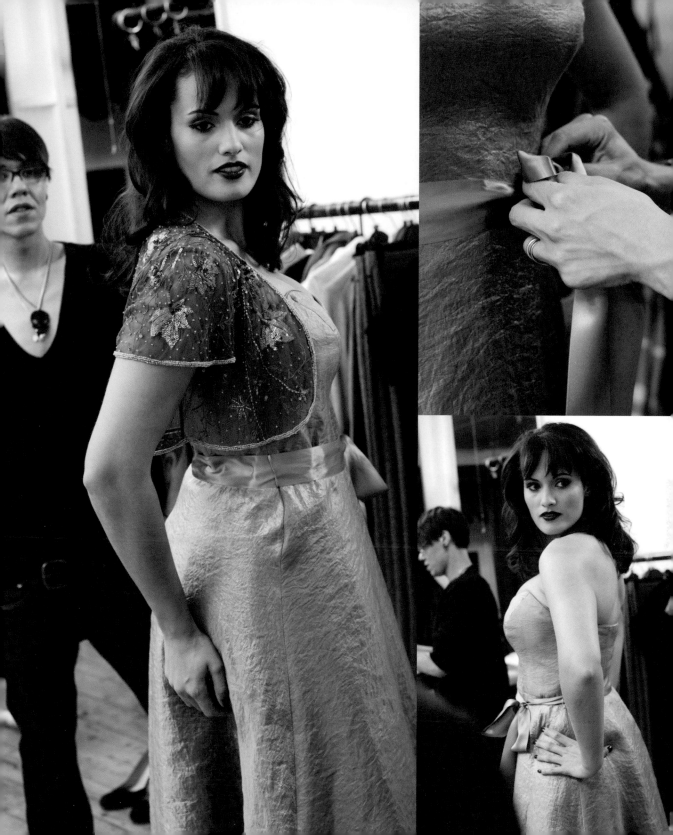

Curvy Girl's Perfect Jackets

Now my gorgeous, because you are curvy, a short fitted jacket will flatter your waist and make your legs look longer. You should be looking out for jackets with panels on the back (then you know it's fitted and shaped). The hem of your jacket should finish just below your tummy to keep it looking trim.

Your best jacket is single-breasted, in a one or two button style, with plenty of chest and collarbone on display. Many jackets have a stitched waistband detail that will keep all eyes on your curves. It's a big old bonus if your jacket also has a belt. That's going to cinch your waist right in (and trust me, your rack is going to look gorgeous).

An open bolero jacket or a knitted shrug is another great option for you, because it will showcase your teeny waist.

STEP AWAY FROM THE RAIL:
- Avoid double-breasted style jackets and those that button up to the neck. They will broaden your top half and make you look like a hotel concierge.

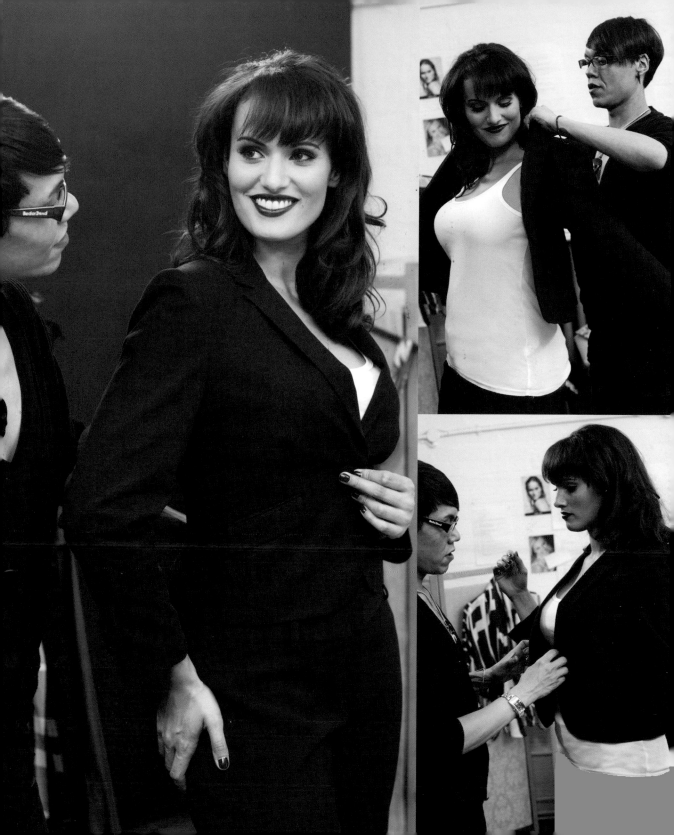

Curvy Girl's Perfect Tops and Skirts

Your perfect skirt is (yes, you guessed it!) a flared or pleated 1950s-style skirt. Like your dream dress, this will skim your hips and thighs while drawing attention to your waist and chest. The skirt should be tailored around your tummy to hold it in, and then flare out over hip and thighs. Hemlines should hit anywhere between your knee or mid calf, depending on how much you love your legs. Steer clear of straight pencil skirts that narrow at the knee will over-exaggerate the roundness of your hips.

For tops and shirts, think corsetry. Look for styles that are fitted from below the chest down to your tummy. Wrap tops are particularly good for this, because they can be adjusted to fit your curves.

STEP AWAY FROM THE RAIL:
- Avoid high-necked blouses and polo-neck knits.
- Also avoid loose, square-cut knits or balloon-shaped smocked tops. These will add bulk, making your top half look huge.

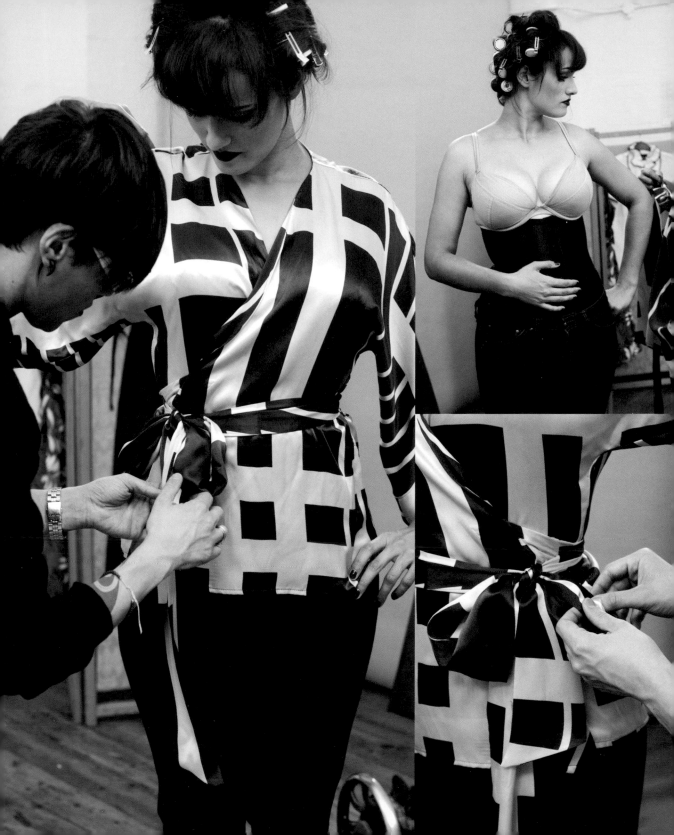

Curvy Girl's Perfect Trousers

If you can't get your hands on diamonds, tailoring is a girl's (next) best friend. There's nothing more chic than womanly curves in a man's suit. But, as always with trousers, it's the cut that counts.

High-waisted wide-legged trousers will skim your lumps and bumps. A wide curved waistband that sits on (not below) your tiny waist will make it the big focus. Look for little darts (vertical half-seams) on the bottom, which will draw your trousers in to skim you at your widest part, before flaring out over your hips and thighs.

Looser, straight-legged (or 'parallel cut') trousers are seriously flattering on your figure. Especially when worn with a short fitted jacket.

SNEAKY STYLING TIP: wearing your trousers a little longer over heels will elongate your legs (and we love that, don't we?).

STEP AWAY FROM THE RAIL:

- Missy, don't think that the best way to make your legs look thinner is to wear the tightest trousers you can squeeze into. Tight or tapered trousers will make your hips and your legs appear wider. (Yes, wider legs. If that doesn't make you run screaming from these styles, nothing will...)

- Cropped trousers will shorten your legs. Unless I'm very much mistaken, no one ever wanted wider, shorter legs...

Curvy Girl's Perfect Shoes

Wherever possible, get some footwear with height, as heels help lengthen your legs. Pointy toes will always be more flattering than round toes, as a longer foot will extend the leg. Try to keep tights and footwear the same colour to streamline your legs. For night, stick to gold or silver shoes that complement your natural skin tone.

STEP AWAY FROM THE RAIL:

- Flat round toed ballet pumps will make your legs look shorter and wider. Did I hear you say "comfortable"?? (are you trying to break my heart??). A pointy shoe with a low kitten heel will be just as easy on the feet. Also; avoid any shoes with ankle straps, which break up the long line of your legs.

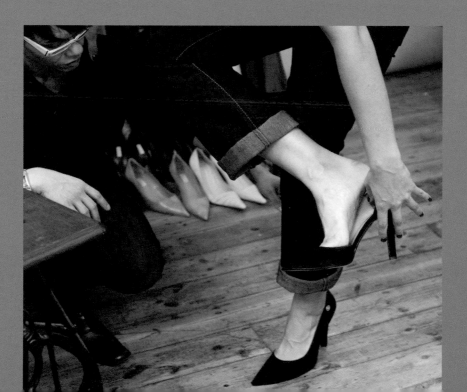

Curvy Girl's Perfect Jeans

Let's face it, jeans shopping is an evil nightmare for everyone. But I know it can be a huge headache for the hourglass honey. Your classic denim dilemma is: fitted waist versus fitted hips. Anything tight enough to fit your waist will crush your hips, and anything that fits your hips will gape at your waistband (helloooo builders' bum).

Unlike with tailored trousers, your best solution is to find a lower-cut waistband that avoids the waist entirely so that you can focus on fitting the hips (and I mean fit: no muffin tops please).

Now, when I say low-cut, I'm not talking about finding the kind of insanely low hipsters that require a new waxing regime. Ideally your waistband should hit just below your belly button. A wide curved waistband will avoid the drafty gap that results in builders' bum. Some jeans have waistbands that are cut higher at the back to avoid you flashing your thong.

Curvy girls should go for classic straight-leg (but not wide) jeans. Also, a darker, uniform-wash denim is more slimming (and more classy) than faded patches and bleached denim.

Again, wear your jeans a little longer over shoes or ankle boots for maximum leg length.

STEP AWAY FROM THE RAIL:

- Exaggerated boot-leg or flared jeans are only flattering on the tallest women.

- Avoid attention-grabbing detailing such as fading, beading, embroidery, etc. around the hip area, unless you are a tweenager or in a girl band.

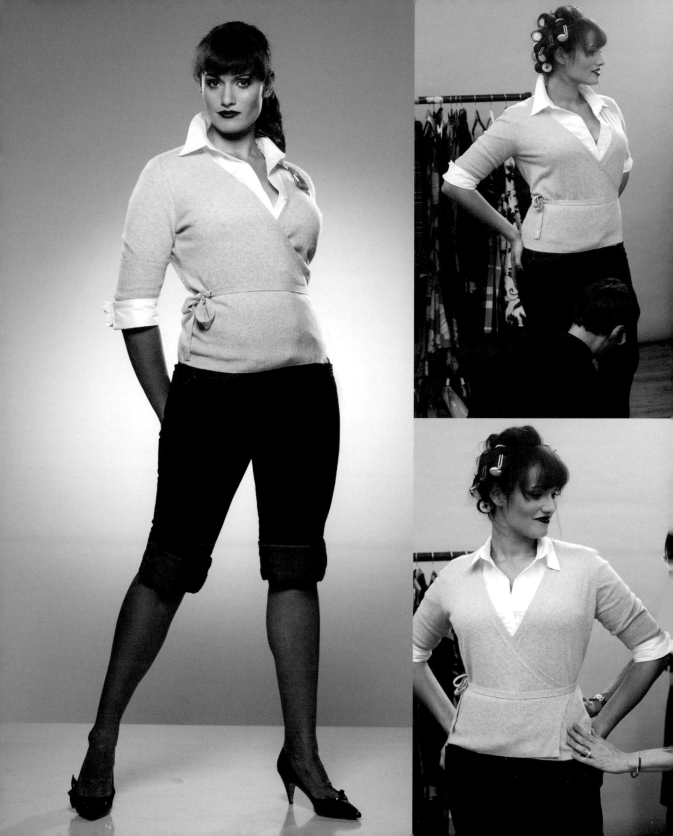

Curvy Girl's Perfect Coats

It's all about the waist again for coats (you still want a foxy silhouette when it's freezing, right?) Keep the collar open and the coat single-breasted, and A-line in shape. (Can you say this in your sleep yet?) Coats with a structured belt are perfect for cinching in, or look out for those featuring a wide stitched waistband detail. Longer, straighter-shaped coats will cover up your killer curves (which would be criminal).

Curvy Girl's Perfect Accessories

A belt is essential for cinching your waist right in. The brighter the better for drawing the eye. Necklaces are also great for highlighting your collarbone (oh, all right then, your hooters...).

STEP AWAY FROM THE RACK:

- Try to avoid belts that are either very wide or ultra-thin, to keep you in perfect proportion.
- Choker-style necklaces and collars will shorten your neck.

Curvy Girl's Rules to Remember

(Repeat after Gok, you little minx...)

- Never try to cover your curves in loose shapes.

- Always keep necklines open.

- Keep the emphasis on your waist with fitted dresses, contrasting belts, and wide waistband-detail stitching on jackets.

- Elongate your legs with loose straight-legged trousers with a high waistband.

- Remember: you are 1950s movie-star glamour personified, my gorgeous!

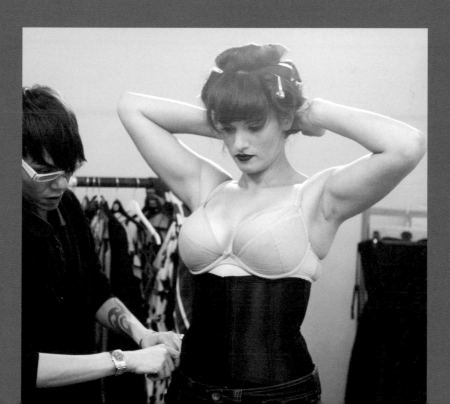

Bellyssimo Babe...

yummy tummies

Let me tell you a secret: guys love women's tummies. There's something about the warm, soft sensuality of your stomach that makes fellas go a little bit loopy. Seriously, it's a big turn-on: there's a reason why the world's oldest dance form is belly dancing...

There are some rare women who naturally have flat or even concave stomachs (FYI: they are nearly always chicks with wider hips). Others do endless sit-ups to get that six pack, while others just push salad around their plates and never eat anything naughty.

I'm hoping that by flagging up the alternatives – wider hips, sit-ups, endless dieting – you might look at your belly with a little more love.

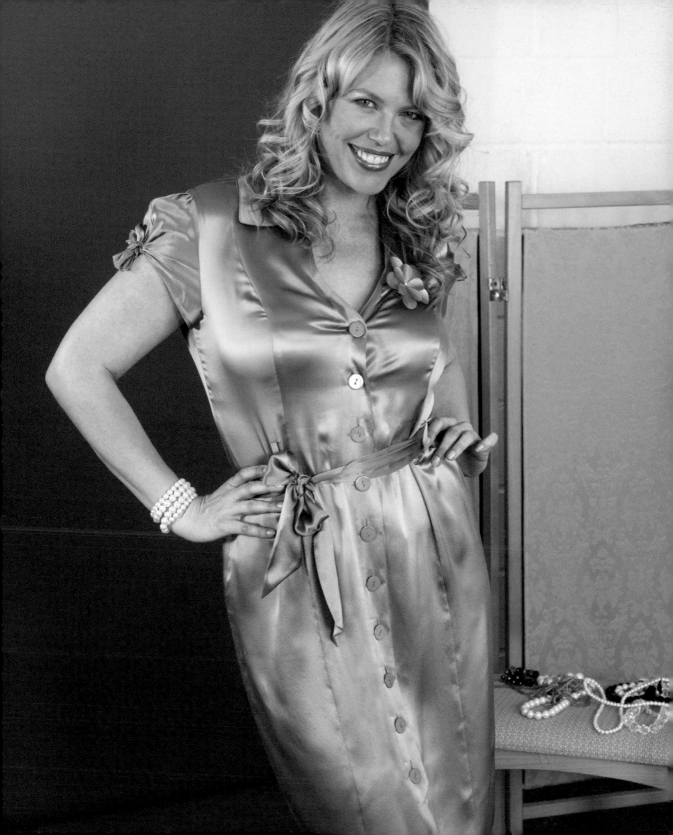

Your Magic Fashion Formula

- Boost boobs.
- Float over your tummy and skim hips.
- Work your waist, legs and arms.

So I want you to know that I think your belly is beautiful. Especially if it shows you've had a baby, or that you like to eat, or that your slinky, skinny hips mean that the bulges have to go somewhere. You are a real woman. And, as I think I've mentioned before, there's a lot to be said for natural beauty.

Four out of five British women wish they weren't as big around their bellies, but you know what? It's a very female thing to focus in on just one part of your body, and miss the bigger picture. It's the overall package that's sexy, my gorgeous. And by obsessively zeroing in on your belly, I bet you frequently forget what most people notice about you: your slim legs, arms, and hips. In short, that you really have an enviable figure.

Let's talk fashion. The most common mistake my bellyssimo babes make is to look for clothes to flatten not flatter. Sneaky tailoring may hold you in, but clingy Lycra won't. For this reason, trousers, skirts and tops should all just graze the crest of your tummy.

Oh, and different clothing brands have different cuts, so don't stubbornly insist on getting your 'usual' size, even though it feels too tight. Go by feel instead, and never fall into the trap of buying trousers that are too tight around the midriff. Buying clothes to fit your skinny hips instead of your stomach will always result in a muffin top.

By the way, everyone needs to know knickers, but particularly you. Adding a pair of magic pants to your wardrobe could literally change your look in an instant. I think you'd be amazed at the results you can achieve from control-top tights or magic knickers. (See Undercover for more info on pain-free tummy tucks.)

But, in the meantime, let's focus on how deceptive dressing can banish those bulges.

Your sexy belly is proof that you like a bit of naughtiness and spice in your life. And you can bet it drives your fella wild!

Bellyssimo Babe's Perfect Dresses

The dress will always be your best friend, for the simple reason that separates will focus in on the very area you are trying to play down: your midriff.

A great way to distract from your belly is to boost your boobs, so that they stick out further than your belly – invest in a great padded or push-up bra! An empire-line dress is perfect for supporting and boosting your chest.

Fabric should never be tight over your tummy. Looser styles can appear shapeless if you don't flash some flesh. Choose body-conscious detailing; such as a feminine V neckline, floaty cap sleeves, and a knee-length hemline, to highlight your legs, arms and chest.

For eveningwear, a neckline that dives into your décolletage will flatter your chest and narrow your torso. Your best dress would be a plunging halter-neck style. But keep that essential empire line silhouette with seaming or a bow tied under the bustline. Make as much use as you can of distracting detailing over your belly: whether it's a vertical panel of pleats to elongate your torso, or side ruching to make your waist look smaller.

For more demure eveningwear, low-waisted dresses can be flattering if you're petite up top, squaring off the whole body to de-emphasize the stomach. If you're a boobilicious babe, a wrap dress is a better bet.

STEP AWAY FROM THE RAIL:

- Silky slip dresses don't have enough detailing to distract from your protruding paunch.
- Bias-cut styles are the queens of cling and will vacuum seal your belly bulge.

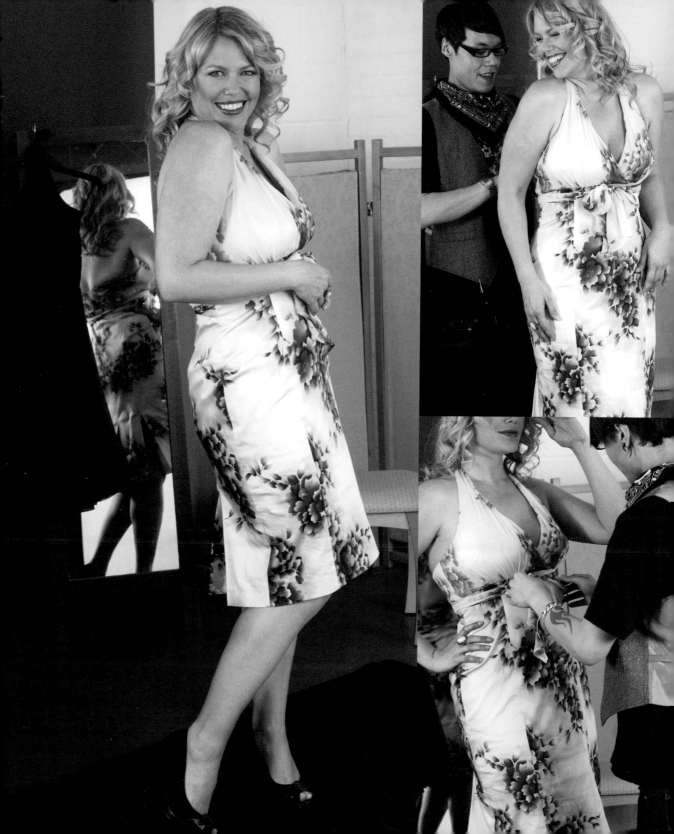

Bellyssimo Babe's Perfect Trousers

Mid-rise trousers (two finger-widths under your belly button) should hit the crest of your tummy, visually bisecting the area. A wider waistband will help hold you in, without cutting into your belly.

Even if you have great legs, avoid skinny styles, which will make your tummy seem larger in comparison. A straight-legged cut will balance you out – and the bigger the belly, the wider your trouser legs should be.

STEP AWAY FROM THE RAIL:

- Avoid drawstring trousers, which will add extra bulk around your midriff. Steer clear of pleats for the same reason.
- Angled pockets will always bag out giving you a saddle-bag silhouette.
- Flat patch pockets on the front of trousers can hide the belly, but even better is to keep the area completely smooth and streamlined by choosing a flat-fronted style with a side zip.

Bellyssimo Babe's Perfect Jackets

Tricksy tailoring is as good as plastic surgery when it comes to body contouring. To reshape your figure, choose a two-button fitted single-breasted jacket that hugs your curves above the waist. The best jacket style for you will have a wide, cinched-in waistband that sits higher than your natural waistline, to elongate your lower body, drawing attention away from your midsection. The hem should then flare out slightly to disguise your stomach, ending at the base of your tummy, to show off your slinky hips and thighs.

Diversion tactics: Interesting lapels will refocus attention away from your midsection: a sexy, satin-lapelled tuxedo jacket is a great example.

STEP AWAY FROM THE RAIL:

- Double-breasted styles will add width to all figures.
- Boxy cropped jackets that end at your waist will just reveal and draw attention to your midsection.

Bellyssimo Babe's Perfect Skirts

Another belly dressing mystery: skirt twisting. Is your waistband constantly revolving? You probably get this with A-line skirts, which are too loose at the hips, then ride up over the curve of your stomach.

The solution: a wide fitted waistband will get your skirt to sit still.

Most flattering on you is a high-waisted pencil skirt, which will work wonders where you least expect it. Choose a style with two darts (tiny vertical seams) below the waistband to smooth out your tummy area.

A hemline that hits the top of the knee will show off your gorgeous legs; and a side split to the thigh can also be really flattering, slicing up the lower body, emphasizing your great legs, and preventing the fabric clinging too tightly at the tummy.

STEP AWAY FROM THE RAIL:

- Skirts with an elasticated waist may be comfortable, but they will also add inches to your midriff (and about twenty years to your perceived age).

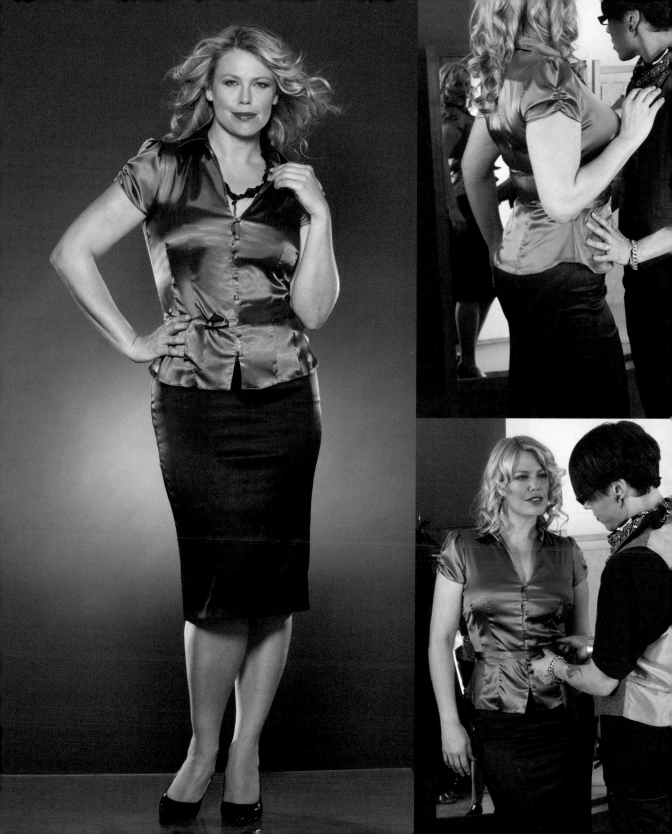

Bellyssimo Babe's Perfect Tops

By now I think you're getting the idea of our tummy trickery: it's all about a figure-skimming empire-line cut – great for boosting the boobs and hiding the belly.

Alternatively, a tailored top with a fitted waist and a softly flared peplum hem will also be very flattering. Cap sleeves can broaden the shoulders, balancing out a thicker midsection. All tops should end at the base of the belly. A lower, more open neckline will break up the area of your upper body, so that there is less focus on your stomach.

Shirts and cardigans can be tricky for you because of straining buttons (never a good look). Your perfect solution: buttonless, wrap-over styles will be far more flattering. These will cinch your waist before flaring out over the stomach (and the end of the tie belt will hang down to distract from your tummy). The V neck will also slice into, and therefore slim, the upper body.

Tops with ruching detailing across the stomach will appear to be hanging loose, which will convince everyone you have a six pack (but don't wear this style skin tight).

STEP AWAY FROM THE RAIL:

- Anything with an elasticated hem will just add more bulk to your midsection.

- Avoid stretchy tops that hug the underside of your belly, emphasizing the curve.

- Longer T-shirts and vests that end mid-thigh will be abruptly interrupted by the bulge of your stomach (think snake swallowing a rodent). Three-quarter-length sleeves that finish at your waist will focus attention on your midriff.

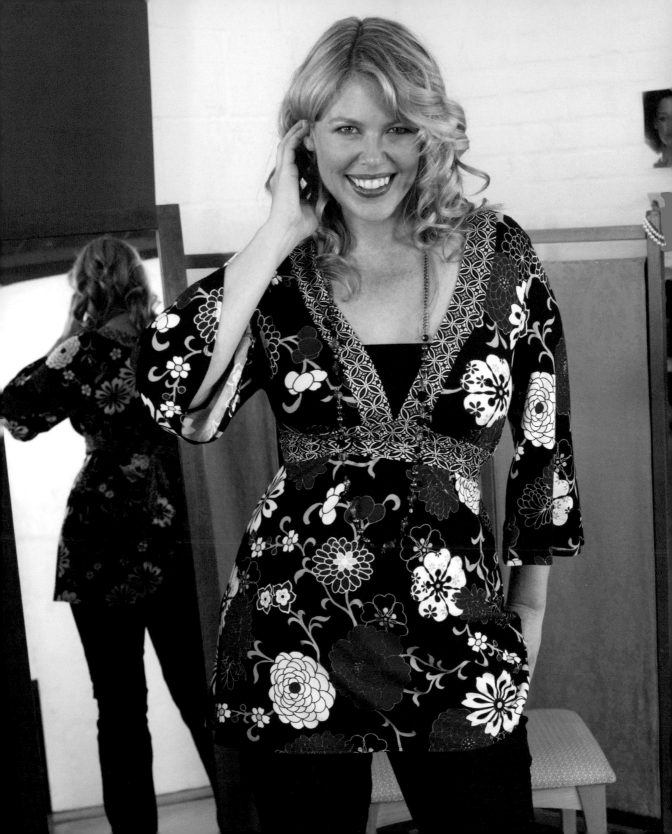

Bellyssimo Babe's Perfect Jeans

Straight-leg, boyish (more square-cut) jeans balance out a heavier mid-section. Go for a mid-rise waistband (again, finishing two finger-widths under the belly button). Alternatively, choose a trouser style with minimal detailing over the tummy. Darker denim will take pounds off you. A crease down each leg will make them look longer and slimmer, as will wearing your jeans with high heels. Look for jeans with a slight stretch (4 per cent Lycra) to cling in all the right places and shape those wobbly bits.

STEP AWAY FROM THE RAIL:

- Avoid ultra-skinny jeans.

- Horizontal 'whisker' fading around the crotch will appear to widen the area around your midriff.

- Ultra-low hipsters may allow you to buy a smaller size (to fit your slim hips) but will also let your love handles hang loose (the dreaded muffin top).

Bellyssimo Babe's Perfect Shoes

Heels will elongate your body, making you look taller and slimmer, while long boots will emphasize great legs. Thigh boots, in case you were wondering, will focus all eyes on your midsection. Chunky heeled, round-toed styles will make your lower body balance better with your midsection than pointy shoes with spiky heels, which may make your silhouette appear to taper down to nothing. Avoid flat shoes as these will always make you look dumpier than wearing heels; go for a kitten heel at least. Steer clear of ankle straps too as they will break up and shorten the line of your legs.

Bellyssimo Babe's Perfect Coats

You want the longer version of your perfect jacket: a high, wide waistband on a single-breasted straight coat will focus on your slim silhouette, and glide over your stomach area. A coat that finishes just above the knee will still show off some leg.

STEP AWAY FROM THE RAIL:

- A belted coat will add bulk to your stomach area.
- Double-breasted styles will appear to broaden your body.
- Cropped styles will focus attention on your tummy.

Bellyssimo Babe's Perfect Accessories

Choose jewellery that draws the eye up to your gorgeous face, such as earrings, corsages and brooches. Chunky bangles will distract from the stomach area. Tying sash belts to one side of your waist will allow the ends to hang down, hiding your stomach. A wide, low-slung belt can cover a smaller potbelly.

STEP AWAY FROM THE RACK:

- Belts worn too tight at the waist will make your stomach bulge outwards even more. Don't make this common big-belly mistake.
- Wide belts will dig into your stomach, and/or ride up your torso.

Everybody has the right to look and feel fabulous ... so no more excuses, hot stuff!

Bellysimo Babe's Rules to Remember

(Repeat after Gok, girlfriend...)

- Don't tuck in tops.

- Avoid Lycra: your clothes should skim, not cling (and never wear anything that's too small).

- Keep skirts and trousers flat-fronted.

- Emphasize your legs and arms by wearing sleeveless and knee-length styles.

- Remember: you are sensual and warm and womanly!

Cleavage Diva...

top heavy and traffic-stopping

One of my favourite images is a 1958 black and white photo of Sophia Loren, caught sneaking an envious glance at Jayne Mansfield's magnificent cleavage as they sit next to each other at dinner. I think it proves that beautiful breasts make men crazy and other women jealous. Even Sophia Loren, whose bronzed (and often Bulgari-strewn) *décolletage* was a wonder to behold.

Maybe this is why British women's breasts are getting bigger, with sales of large bra sizes tripling over the last three years.

The average bra size in the UK is now 36C, up from 34B a decade ago, and an estimated 40 per cent of women take a D cup or above. Bravo, ladies!

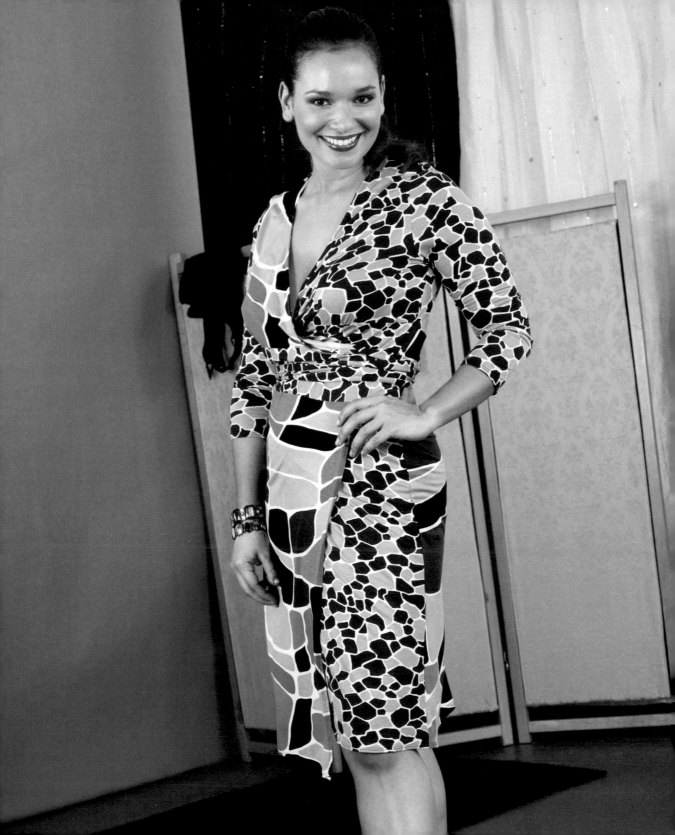

Your Magic Fashion Formula

- Open necklines.

- Low waistbands.

- Tops that skim the ribcage and hips.

- Gentle A-line and boot-cut styles to balance the silhouette.

But not everyone believes that bigger necessarily means better. An estimated 4000 British women have breast reductions each year, because of the physical, practical or psychological problems that sometimes go with having a larger chest.

Fashion-wise, a great rack can either make or break an outfit. Hiding your breasts in baggy shapeless tops will add pounds to you; whereas if your top is too tight your look instantly goes tarty.

You need structure to show off your curves. You will also have to face the fact that your fantastic rack may make buying clothes off-the-rail a bit tricky. If you've got a tiny waist and massive hooters, alterations are going to make all the difference to an outfit.

Of course, the main challenge with major cleavage is looking tastefully sexy. I've styled loads of glamour models for shoots over the years (I love those ladies), so believe me: I understand about playing up your assets without letting them take over (clue: when men can't look you in the face, your breasts are too in-your-face).

Frustratingly for you, it really is a fine line between sensual and Slutsville. Try to avoid anything too tight or short on your bottom half, and flash some collarbone to offset your assets. My best advice to you is that your breasts are better showcased by cleavage rather than girth. Surprisingly: better a demure hemline than a demure neckline.

BEST FRIEND ADVICE: Never hide behind your boobs. Your personality is more than your chest.

A gorgeous cleavage can be a major style statement, but you need to know how to showcase your assets.

Cleavage Diva's Perfect Dresses

It's hard for chesty chicks to find dresses that will fit both their top and bottom halves. One option is to find a dress that fits your biggest measurement – your chest – and then have it taken in from the bust-line down. Or, two-piece outfits in the same fabric may help you find the best fit.

Big breasts can make you appear to be big all over, so try body skimming styles that show off your slimmest bits. Open vertical necklines will highlight your neck and collarbone, and fitted shapes will hug your ribcage.

Top-heavy girls can often seem shorter, so elongating your body is essential. A V-neck will help with this. Empire-line styles with horizontal seaming under your bust will make your body seem longer.

A dress with an A-line skirt, with a hemline finishing just below the knee, will be the best shape to balance out your breasts without adding bulk. For those with great arms, an A-line V-neck shift is a great style to focus on your slimmest bits. A wrap dress, in a stiffer fabric to give less cling over the bust, and with a more A-line shape, could be a good alternative.

Three-quarter-length sleeves will draw attention to your slim waist. Long, loose sleeves with a tapered or flared cuff will pull the focus away from your chest. Choose wider straps on sleeveless styles to support and balance out your bust (and hide a bra).

STEP AWAY FROM THE RAIL:

- Very wide horizontal necklines, like slash or boat necks, or off-the-shoulder styles, will broaden the shoulders, making you seem more top-heavy.

- Short sleeves will direct all eyes to bust level.

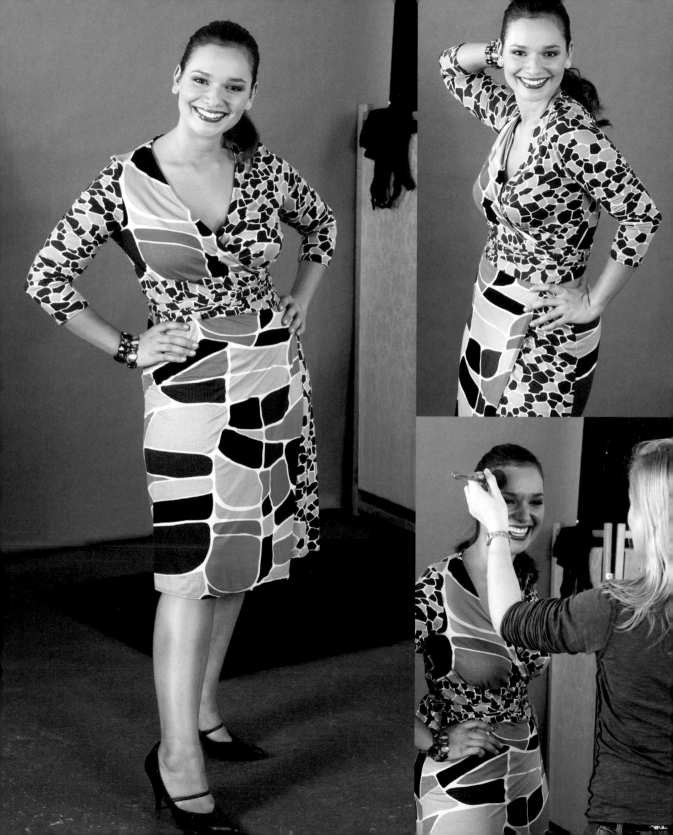

Cleavage Diva's Perfect Eveningwear

For evening, apply the same rules as for daytime dresses, but rack up the glamour factor with slinky fabrics and eye-catching colours. A torso-clinging V-neck empire-line dress, with a soft A-line skirt and inverted pleats at the hem, ticks all the right boxes.

Never go braless. Find a dress that can accommodate support (or, as in some designer dresses, has support built in). Hunt down plunge bras with clear front straps, and convertible strap styles. A one-shoulder dress is a good compromise, flashing some flesh but still allowing you to wear a convertible (one-strap) bra.

Any kind of detailing at the bust will just focus attention to that area, so keep it simple. Draping at the neckline will add bulk to your breasts. (Besides, 'draping' is a fancy word for 'drooping', so it may give the impression of sagginess.)

STEP AWAY FROM THE RAIL:

- Straight styles will direct all eyes up to the bust.
- Loose styles that hang from the chest can make you look cube-shaped.
- High-neck styles can make you look matronly.
- Avoid low necklines unless they are bra-friendly.
- Strapless or backless numbers, and dresses with thin straps, won't accommodate sufficient support.

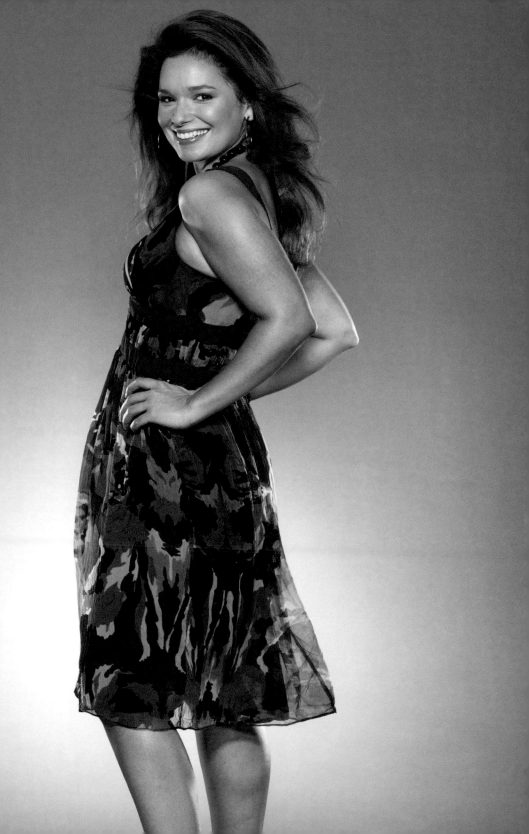

Cleavage Diva's Perfect Jackets

When you have a large chest it automatically broadens your torso, which can make you look short-waisted. So it is important to lengthen your body line with some nifty tailoring.

Your perfect jacket will be softly shaped rather than tightly tailored, to complement, rather than exaggerate, your curves. A low-cut jacket, buttoning under the bust-line and gently fitted at the ribcage, will slice into your torso, elongating your upper body. A longer-line jacket that finishes beneath the belly will also add length. Steer clear of any styles that button higher than your bust-line, which will make your breasts appear bigger.

Strong structured or puffed shoulders can make the chest seem smaller in comparison, as can long, fitted sleeves, with a slight flare at the cuff. Long, narrow lapels will slim down your breasts.

Add subtle volume to the hips with pockets or embellishment, to make the waist appear smaller, and balance the size of the chest. Lightweight stretch fabrics can give you a sleeker fit and will streamline your silhouette.

SNEAKY STYLING TIP: Watch out for jackets (and other garments) with 'princess seaming'. These vertical seams curve through the centre of each breast, then down the ribs, forming a chunky Y-shape on your torso. Not only does princess seaming improve the fit, but the Y-shape effectively draws a slimmer silhouette onto your upper body. Brilliant!

SNEAKY STYLING TIP: Leaving a fitted jacket undone can visually break up the bust-line, leaving just a slim central panel of clothing visible beneath, to elongate the body.

STEP AWAY FROM THE RAIL:

- Boxy square-cut jackets will obscure any waist definition.
- Avoid wearing large patterns or a lighter colour on top than that on your bottom half. Large lapels will add weight to the chest.
- Avoid thick, heavy fabrics, like tweed or fur or bouclé, which will add extra inches.
- Belted styles will look too severely cinched, exaggerating the size of your breasts.
- Shoulder pads will just increase upper body bulk.

Cleavage Diva's Perfect Trousers

Trousers can be tricky for you. The frustration with top-heavy figures is that highlighting those slinky hips and your tiny tush will just make your chest look even bigger. Leg width is the key here: you want wider trousers that skim the hips.

A lower waistband will elongate the torso, refocusing the attention away from the chest. Wearing lighter colours or a subtle pattern will balance you out and draw the eye down and away from the chest. Belts, pockets and detailing across the front will all help add volume to the hips.

STEP AWAY FROM THE RAIL:

- High-waisted trousers will shorten and broaden your upper body, turning your chest into a shelf.

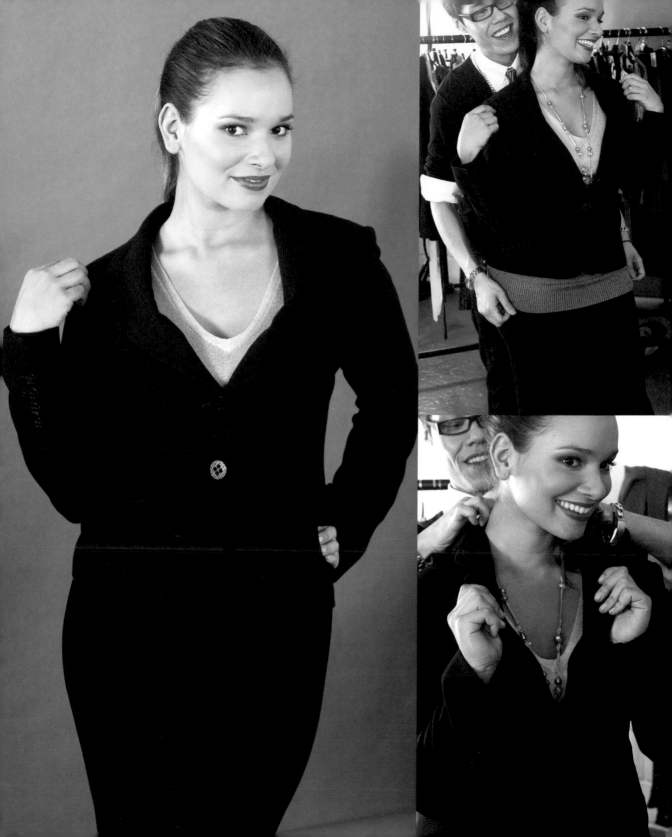

Cleavage Diva's Perfect Skirts

Your ideal hem length to balance out those hooters is on or below the knee (so you can still show off a bit of leg). A-line shapes, or a straighter style with a bit of flippy flare at the hem, will add subtle volume to your lower half, to set off the width of your chest.

Interesting hems will draw the eye down, making the legs appear longer, and giving them some attention. A lower waistband will elongate the torso.

STEP AWAY FROM THE RAIL:

- Looking leggy and booby is probably overkill, so avoid short skirts, however great your legs.

- As with trousers, a high waistband will sit beneath your chest like a shelf.

- Straight skirts will draw the eye straight up to the chest.

- Very wide gathered or pleated styles will just add bulk, making you appear larger all over.

- Never wear black on your bottom half (even if you're wearing black on top). Your legs will seem miniscule compared to your chest.

Cleavage Diva's Perfect Tops

Deep V necklines will divide your breasts and lengthen the vertical line of your upper body. Fine knits, T-shirts and waist-fitting wrap tops will all cling to your curves. Other great vertical necklines are sweetheart or low scoop-neck.

Shirts have that essential V-neck but are trickier to fit to your curves. If necessary, buy a shirt that fits your chest, then have it taken in on the ribcage.

Longer sleeves flatter a large chest. Three-quarter-lengths will focus attention on the waist, and sleeveless styles will highlight slim arms. Avoid short sleeves that end at chest level as they will focus attention on your boobs.

Waistcoats can be very flattering for toning down a large chest, as they break up the vertical line of the torso. Traditional styles have a mini buckled strap for waist-cinching. The pointed hemline will emphasise the hips.

We all know black is more slimming, but feeling like you always have to wear it is very restricting. Just be sure that your top is darker and plainer than your bottom half.

STEP AWAY FROM THE RAIL:

- Horizontal stripes will widen your chest, but also avoid vertical stripes, which will just exaggerate the curve of your breasts.

- Looser weave knits will make your chest look as if it's straining at the fabric.

- Short puff sleeves are also a no no as they will echo your breasts, like four balloons in a row.

- High necklines such as polo-necks will make you appear buxom.

- Cropped styles will make your waist look smaller, but your chest bigger as will very tight sweaters.

- Fussy detailing over your boobs – pockets, prints, ruffles – will exaggerate your chest.

Cleavage Diva's Perfect Shoes

Pointy-toed shoes will work well with wide-leg trousers. Chunky heeled boots will balance out your boobs, and are good for breaking up the line of the leg. Furry flat boots over jeans are a great look for winter, evening out your silhouette.

STEP AWAY FROM THE RACK:
- Avoid delicate shoes, like very high strappy sandals or high-heeled ankle boots, which will taper your silhouette down into a cone shape.

Shoes are like sex: you can never have enough.

Cleavage Diva's Perfect Accessories

A low-slung belt will accentuate and broaden the hips. A big bag worn at hip level, or a large tote carried down by your side, will balance out your silhouette. Also, keep jewellery at hip level, such as chunky rings and bangles.

STEP AWAY FROM THE RACK:

- Avoid corsages, brooches, etc., which will focus all attention on the breasts.

- Long necklaces will appear to be hanging off a precipice, while chokers and scarves worn at the neck will crowd the neckline, adding bulk.

- A small bag worn tucked under the arm will be dwarfed by your frontbags!

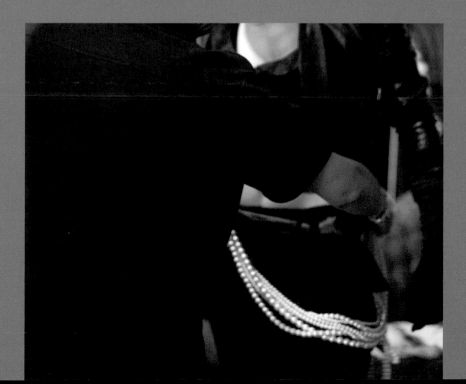

Cleavage Diva's Perfect Jeans

A perky, denim-clad bottom is a great way to add volume, without bulk, and to balance out your bust. You want straight jeans with a mid-width leg. Hipster jeans will, like a lower waistband on trousers, elongate your torso and make you appear taller.

Choose detailing like front pockets to emphasize the hips, and higher-set flap pockets on the backside to perk up flat buttocks. A lighter-wash denim, with some bleaching on the thighs or whiskered fading across the stomach, will also add subtle volume to the lower half.

Wearing your jeans slightly longer with heels will help give the impression of a longer body line, which de-emphasizes your chest.

STEP AWAY FROM THE RAIL:

- Darker washes and skinny styles will make your lower half look slimmer, and your body even more top-heavy.

- Boot-cut jeans that are tight at the knees will also over-emphasize your chest.

- Be careful when finding your perfect cut: you want a mid-width jean, not a baggy one.

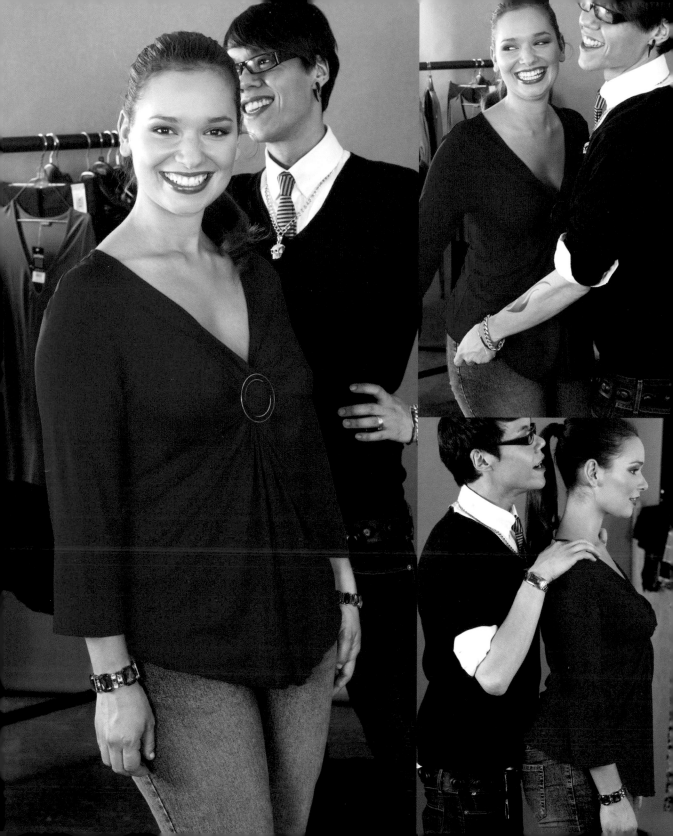

Cleavage Diva's Perfect Coats

Avoid the problem of not being able to find a coat you can close over your chest by looking for a style with a wide, open neck. Again, go for narrow lapels to avoid 'choking' the neck area. Instead, choose a one-button style (or concealed buttons) that fastens under the bust-line. Raised empire-line seaming, or high-waisted 1940s tailored styles, flatter fuller chests as they emphasize slim hips. Look for soft A-line shapes finishing below the knee. Large flap pockets on the hips will also be great for balancing your figure.

STEP AWAY FROM THE RAIL:

- Avoid double-breasted styles, which broaden your chest.
- Rows of buttons will accentuate the curve of your chest.
- Furry collars will just add bulk.

Cleavage Diva's Rules to Remember

(Repeat after Gok, girlfriend…)

- Never wear loose tops: they should be fitted beneath your bust-line.

- Always keep necklines open.

- Keep bottoms low-waisted, lighter or patterned, and flared or boot-cut at the hem.

- Empire-line dresses will lengthen your torso.

- Don't forget: Tastefully sexy.

Slim and Sexy...

skinny and fabulous

Hello! Can you say 'born lucky'?

So you're tall and thin, which are the to-die-for supermodel proportions, and the 41 per cent of British women who are constantly on a diet hate you!

Now, being the shape of the moment, you should feel body-confident to the point of smugness, right? But so many skinny women don't feel sexy or feminine: they are too busy worrying that they're gawky and awkward and boyish.

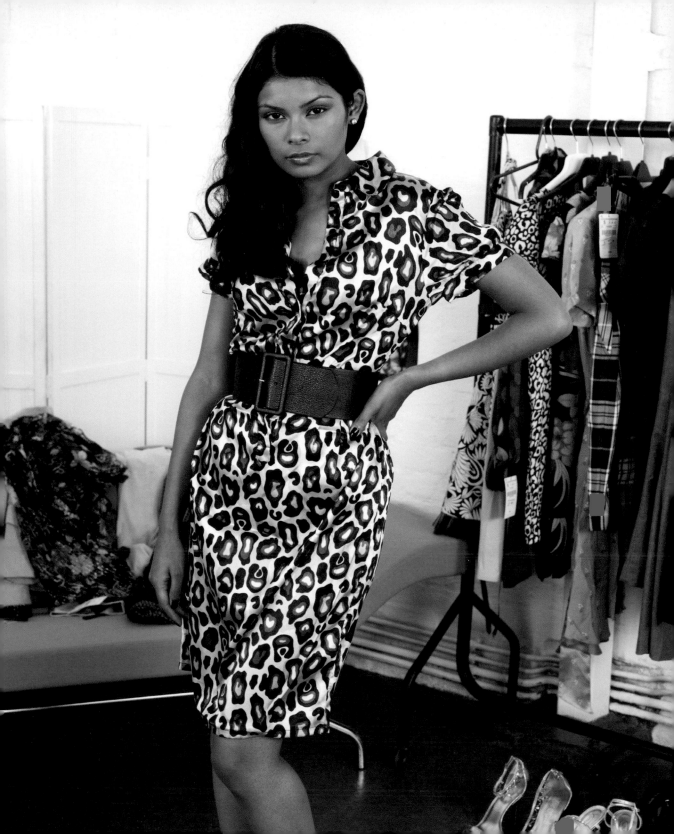

Your Magic Fashion Formula

- Cinch the waist.
- Add volume at the hips and chest with pleats and gathers.

The big issue? You all want bigger bazookas! I still love supermodel Naomi Campbell's claim that the perfect breast can fit inside an old-fashioned shallow champagne glass – though of course, she's biased. Besides, I've never met a girl who wasn't in love with Audrey Hepburn, or a guy who doesn't fancy Kate Moss or Keira Knightley. So let's agree that your mini-boobs are elegant, cool, sexy, feminine and classy.

Being tall and thin, there is a long list of clothes that you can wear, but I want to focus specifically on styles that will make you look curvaceous. Personally, I think a statuesque willowy woman in a clingy, slit-to-the navel dress looks stunning. But it won't give her curves. And if you want curves, my gorgeous, Gok's gonna give you CURVES!

Of course, clothes have got to fit. This might seem like an obvious point, but for skinny girls this is especially important. Clothes that are too tight will make you look even skinnier. Most people want to achieve this effect, but if you are über thin, maybe you don't.

I can't make you look like you're 36DD, but I can promise to stop you looking 2D. The key to doing this is simple: keep clothes 3D, with curved seaming and volume detailing, all of which will add depth to your outfits, and a little cha-cha-cha to your chest.

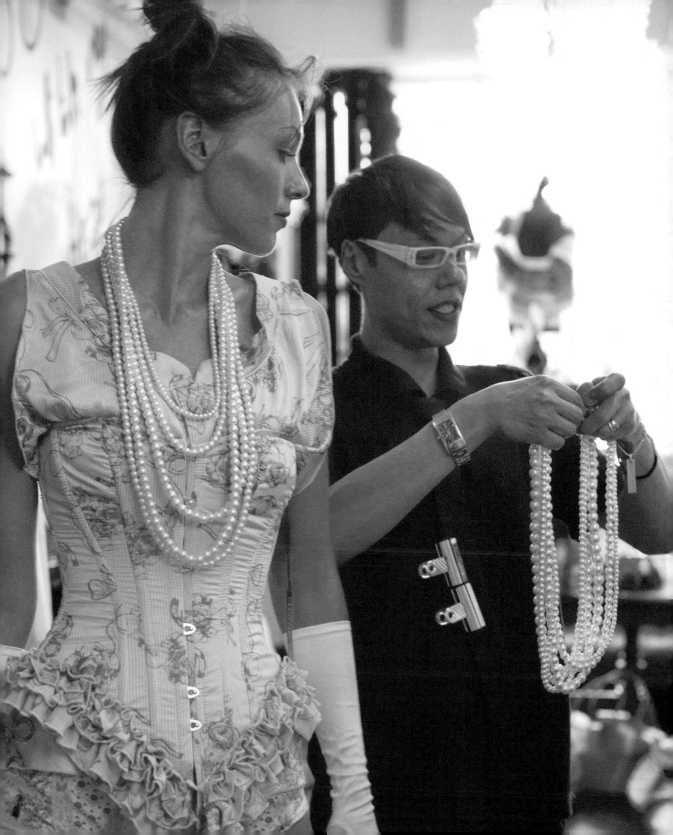

Slim Girl's Perfect Dresses

Forget implants, but let's use a bit of nip and tuck in your wardrobe. You want curvier hips and a chest, and a carved-out waist? The easiest way to achieve this is with nifty tailoring details: curved seaming and contrast piping will act as body contouring, drawing on the figure you really want. Meanwhile, smartly placed gathering or excess detailing like ruffles will create fullness over the bust and hips.

Slim ladies should always look for a dress with 'hanger appeal'. I don't want to spook you, but does that dress look like it's already got a body inside it while it's still on the hanger? That's the dress for you. Has it already got volume at the chest and hips, a wide fitted waistband or a tightly cinched-in waist? Basically, if the dress already has better curves than you do, buy it.

Keep necklines as high as possible for added curves, and soften thin limbs with puff or cap sleeves.

For day, a patterned cap-sleeved shirt dress, with flap breast and hip pockets, belted at the waist, is a smart option. The excess detailing will add shape where you need it, while the belt will cinch your waist to emphasise your hips and chest.

STEP AWAY FROM THE RAIL:

- Stretchy wrap dresses need curves. This is one garment that always looks better on 'real people' than catwalk models.

- Avoid any garment with zero 'hanger appeal'. Empire-line styles will make your legs look a hundred miles long.

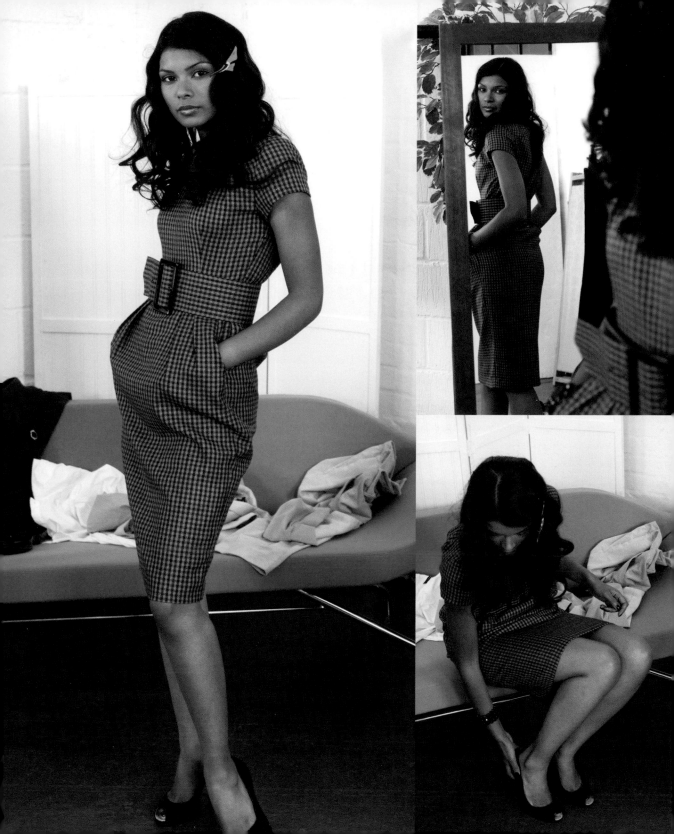

Slim Girl's Perfect Eveningwear

Some skinny girls have a real complex about eveningwear. They worry that the less they wear, the more angular they look.

To soften your shape, high-tied halter-necks with vertical gathers across the chest are an elegant look and will create fullness. High necklines will add interest to your chest area. A low, softly draped back can add width to your body's profile.

Boost that bottom with dresses with a flared or gathered skirt, which will add volume and emphasize your waist. Or try a bubble-shaped skirt, tapered in at the waist and hem, to give you curvy hips.

Black is slimming, so you should avoid plain black dresses. To give you a greater physical presence, try dresses that are multicoloured, whether it's an eye-catching large print or a dress with different colour-blocked sections to chop up the body and add interest. Light-reflecting or shiny fabrics will be very flattering on you, softening your silhouette.

STEP AWAY FROM THE RAIL:

- Ultra-slim babes should try to avoid styles that reveal their boniest areas: from a deep V that extends below the chest, to strapless styles that focus on the shoulders.

- Avoid skin-tight plain tops that will draw attention to your flat chest. On a flat chest, corsets will look like armour-plating.

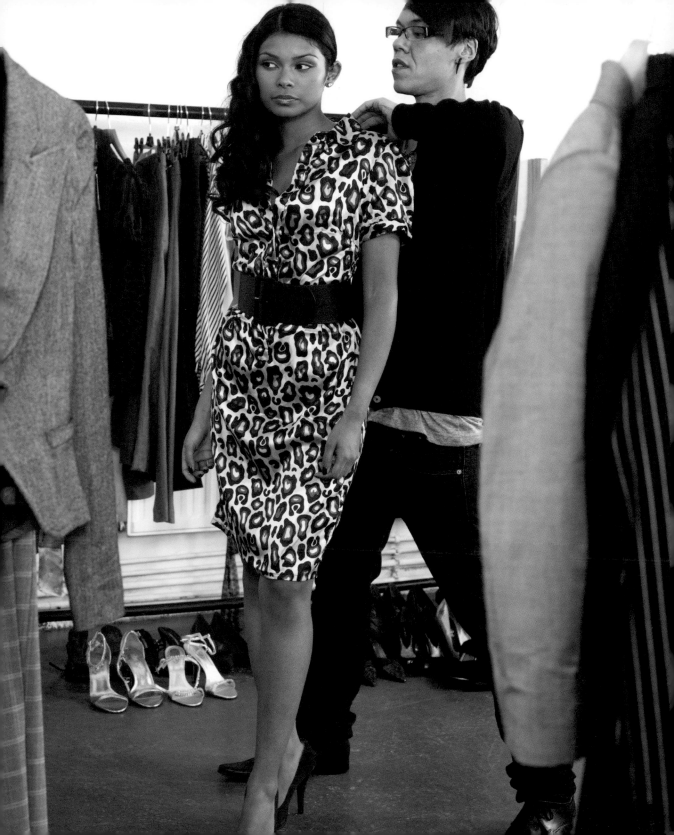

Slim Girl's Perfect Trousers

Masculine tailoring gives *vive la différence* sexy sophistication to a slim lady. Build up the volume with wide trousers featuring pleats, patch pockets and turn-ups.

Thick and busy fabrics such as plaid or tweed will give you a greater visual presence. Cuffed pleated knee-length shorts are a funky alternative, worn with knee-high boots. Stay well away from pinstripes as these will elongate your frame to make you look even taller and thinner, as will very narrow trousers or stretch styles with no detailing.

Slim Girl's Perfect Jackets

Bulk up in boxy jackets in leather or fake fur, or a tailored jacket with seaming at the chest, waist and hips, to add curves and depth. Any jacket with a tightly fitted and/or belted waist and structured shoulders is good for body contouring. Breast and hip pockets will also add volume.

STEP AWAY FROM THE RAIL:
- An outsized, double-breasted masculine blazer is a great look on a skinny chick, but its bagginess will emphasize your lack of curves.

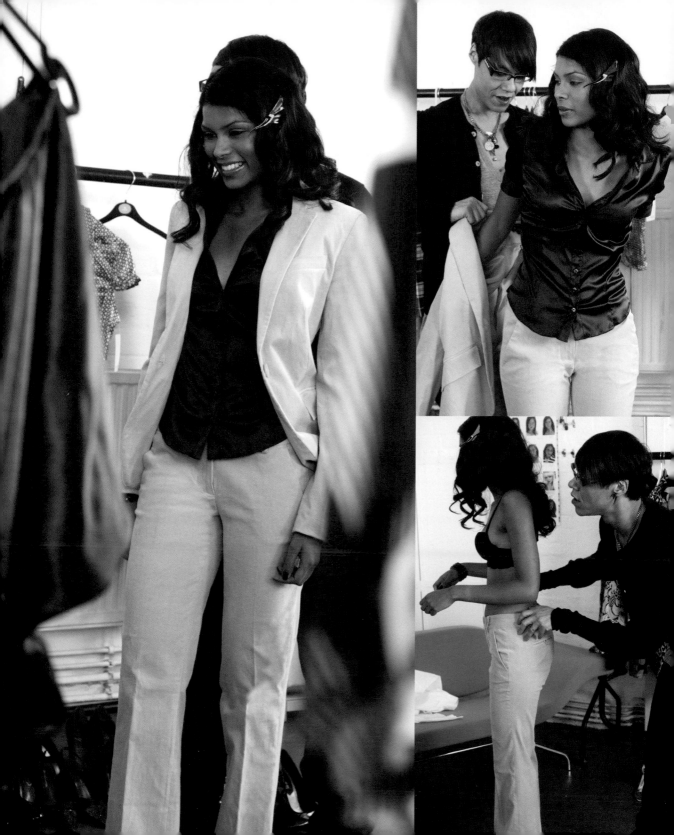

Slim Girl's Perfect Tops

Your rule for tops: if it's flat, forget it!

To max your rack you want ruching, smocking, ruffles and gathers across the chest to make the area look bigger. A pussy-bow, puff-sleeved blouse in a floaty fabric will give you maximum volume, especially one with large cuffs and collars. A cinched waist with a peplum hem will carve out an hourglass shape. Or layer under a waistcoat or knitted sleeveless tank top for curve-creating depth.

A crisp cotton shirt can give you as much structure as a jacket: look for a fitted waist, breast flap-pockets and wide collars. A slash-neck horizontal striped top is a great optical illusion to broaden your chest and shoulders.

STEP AWAY FROM THE RAIL:

- Lose the Lycra. Any skin-tight top or fine knit will cling to (and over-emphasize) your flat chest.

- A plain, skinny-cut T-shirt will turn you 2D.

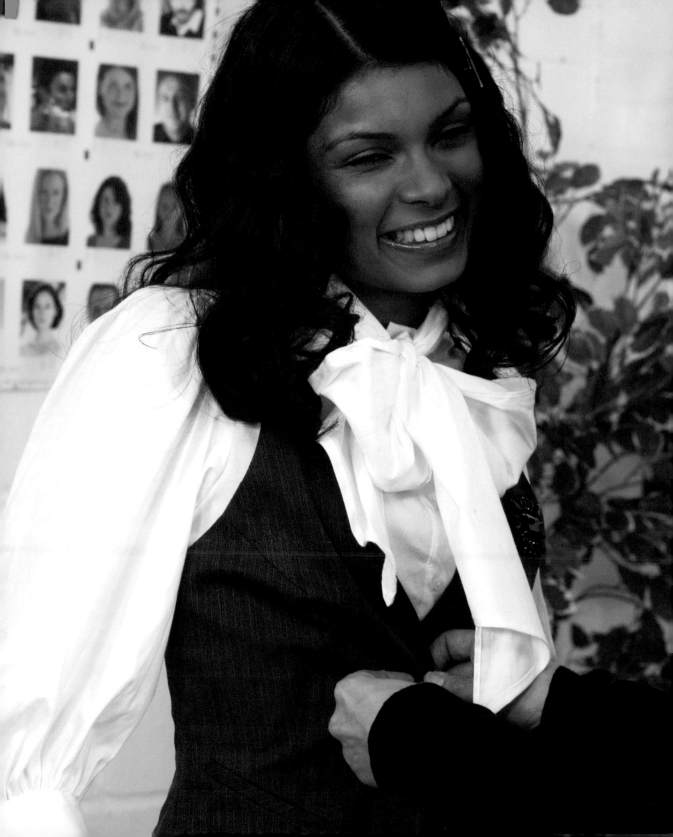

Slim Girl's Perfect Skirts

Once again, we're looking for volume. A full skirt defines the waist, creating an hourglass shape. Hemlines ending below the knee will make your calves look curvier. Wearing your hems higher than knee-length will show off your enviably thin legs, but will also make you look less curvaceous. Sharp A-line shapes will make legs look like shoelaces, so go for a pencil skirt that narrows at the hem (especially if it then kicks out again into pleats or frills). This will make your hips appear rounder.

Slim Girl's Perfect Accessories

Load on long necklaces to create depth and interest at your chest. Or use a silk scarf tied around the neck to soften your look. You can carry off a gigantic bag with style.

STEP AWAY FROM THE RACK:
- Avoid big bangles, which will make your arms look like sticks. A cuff or chain bracelet would be more proportionate.
- Avoid tiny bags, which will make you seem like a giant in comparison.

Slim Girl's Perfect Shoes

Round toes, ankle straps and ankle boots will all crop the length of your legs, and emphasize your calves, making them look curvier. Flat ballet pumps are chic with skirts or trousers and can soften your look. Round-toed flat riding boots worn over jeans will break up your legs and create curves. Don't be afraid of patterned tights: you can totally carry them off, and they will add width to your legs.

STEP AWAY FROM THE RACK:

- Avoid pointy-toed shoes with spiky high heels, which will elongate your legs and make you appear more angular.
- Stretch boots will cling unflatteringly to thin legs, while boots that are too loose for your calves will just emphasise your skinniness.

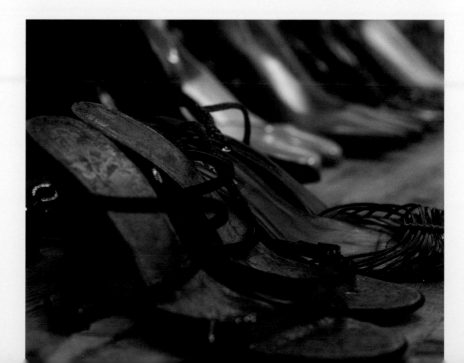

Slim Girl's Perfect Jeans

Low-waisted, straight-legged boy-cut jeans are really flattering for slim hips. Choose a stiff or soft but thicker denim. Subtle shading on the thighs will add shape to your legs. Choose flap pockets at the front or back to add volume – pockets that are angled or higher will lift the bottom. Jeans should touch the bottom of the ankle bone, or tuck them into long boots to create shape for your legs. Always wear a contrasting belt to emphasize your hips. Higher-waisted jeans will also emphasize the curve of your bum and waist.

STEP AWAY FROM THE RAIL:
- Boot-cut jeans just look flat on taller women.
- Skinny stretch jeans will make your legs look even skinnier.

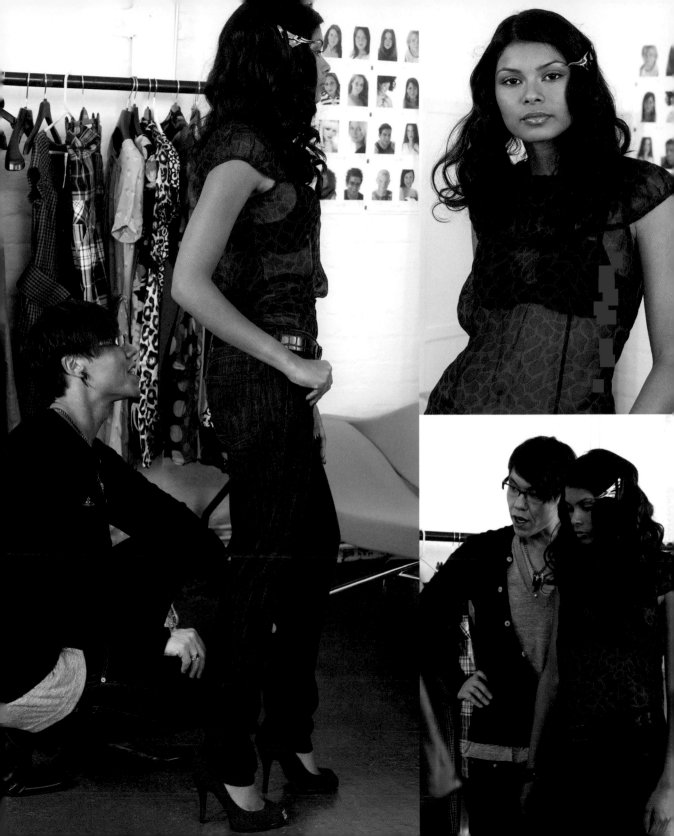

Slim Girl's Perfect Coats

As demonstrated by Audrey Hepburn herself, a classic double-breasted trench coat has exactly the kind of excess detailing that you're looking for – epaulettes, shoulder flaps, belts, buttons and buckles – to create volume while still emphasising the waist.

STEP AWAY FROM THE RAIL:

- A slim-fit straight-cut Crombie-style coat will make you look slimmer and straighter.

- An unstructured 'edge to edge' coat will just hang off you.

Slim Girl's Rules to Remember

(Repeat after Gok, you sexy thing...)

- Don't buy flat clothes: go for ruffles, ruching, gathers and volume and structure of any kind.

- Avoid plain black. Use print, colour and shiny fabrics to soften your silhouette.

- Know your size. Clothes that are skin-tight or too baggy will make you look skinny.

- Excess detailing like curved seaming or piping will contour your body.

- Look for clothes with a squarer cut: e.g. boxy jackets or boy-cut jeans.

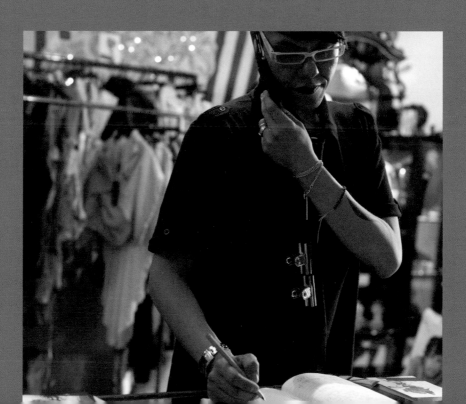

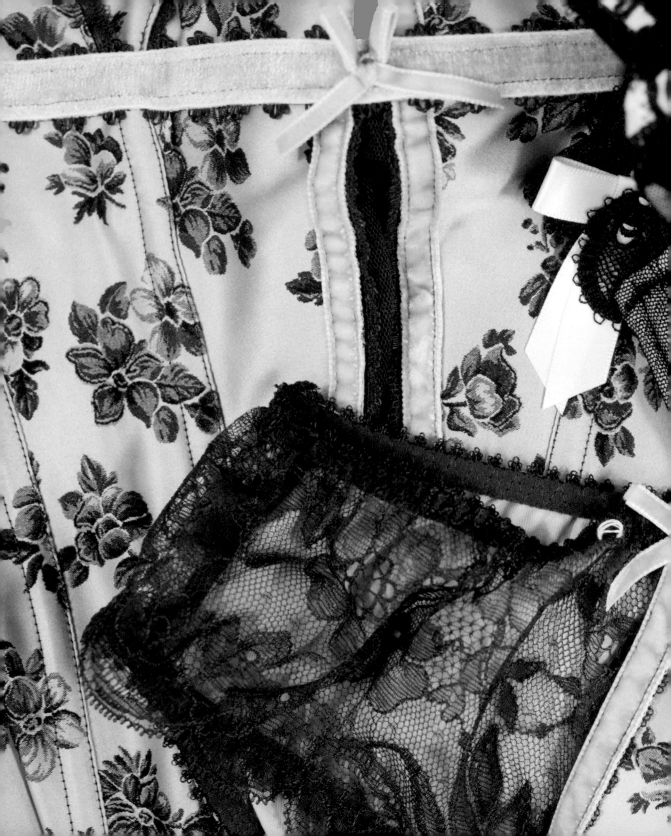

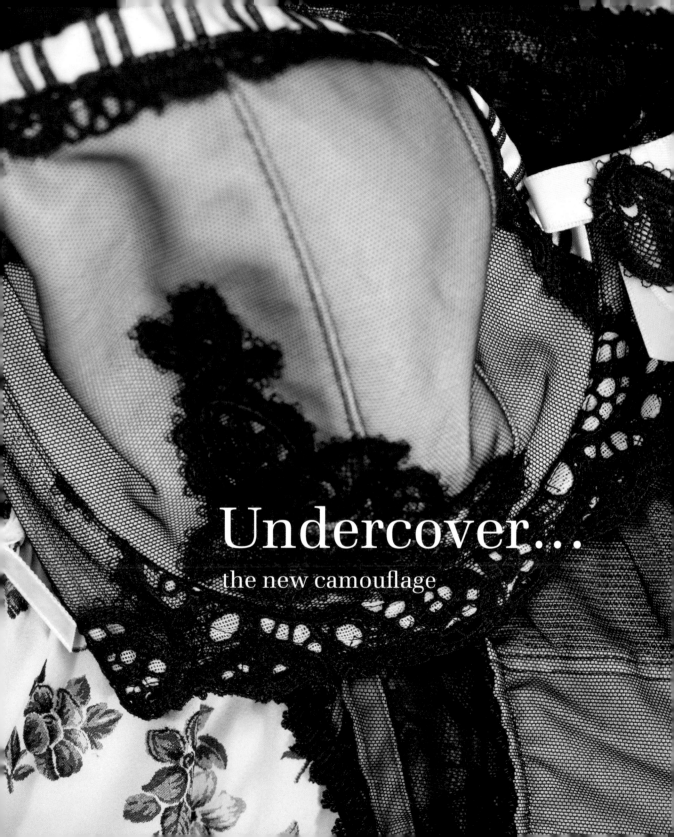

Undercover...

the new camouflage

In this chapter I'm going to show you how to use underwear to showcase that beautiful body of yours in the best possible way, by enhancing your natural shape.

Gorgeous lingerie is, of course, a great mood-enhancer. It's all about self-indulgence, being ultra-feminine, and having the self-confidence that comes from knowing you are wearing something beautiful that only you can see.

Proper underwear does in seconds what surgery takes months and big money to achieve – uplifting, streamlining, and nipping in.

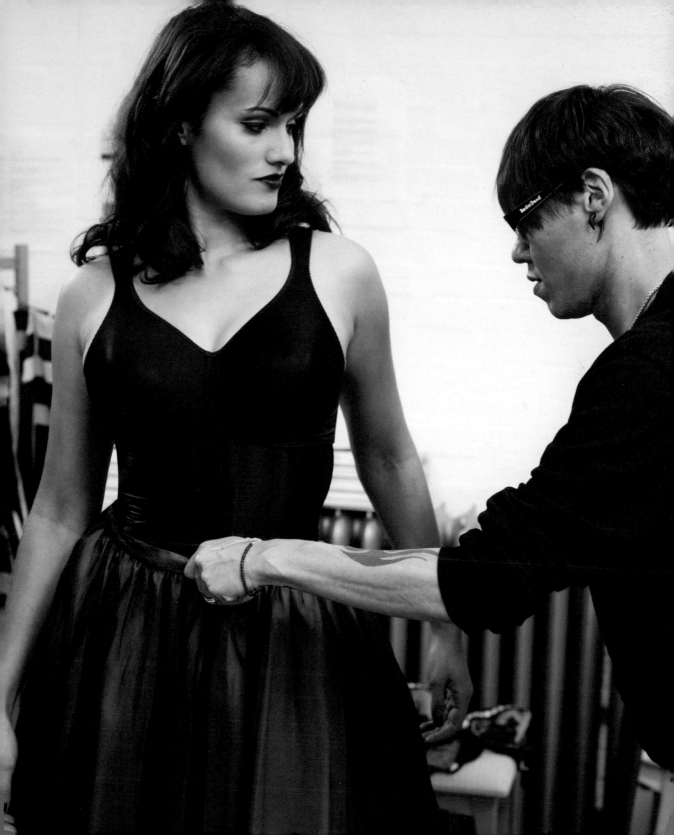

Good lingerie is one of the simple (daily!) pleasures in life, so why would you want to miss out?

Conversely, nothing will make you feel less pleased with your naked body than schlumping around in nasty greying baggy underwear! (If I had my way, all multi-pack cotton bikini briefs would be burnt.) Just think: that saggy underwear is probably making you look saggier than you actually are! (*Do you want to look saggier? Seriously...*)

From talking to my ladies, I know that the main reason for underwear neglect is thinking that it can't be seen, so therefore it doesn't matter. Well, think again. Rubbish underwear is very visible: from saggy bikini briefs under tight trousers or skirts, to too-tight lingerie under fitted dresses and bumpy lace bras under T-shirts. Bad underwear will ruin any outfit and every bedroom striptease (in short, it will crucify all your steamy sessions!).

I really believe it's better to live in a simple T-shirt and jeans with excellent shapely underwear than to have amazing designer clothes with floppy unsupported lumps and bumps underneath. Better to cancel your gym membership and spend the money on your perfect underwear. I mean it! The right-sized underwear can literally make you look like a new woman.

Seven out of ten British women think their lives would be improved if they had a better body. Well, gorgeous, now is your chance to find out...

Good underwear can take you down at least one dress size, and the correct bra or magic knickers can massively increase your options for clothes that suit your body.

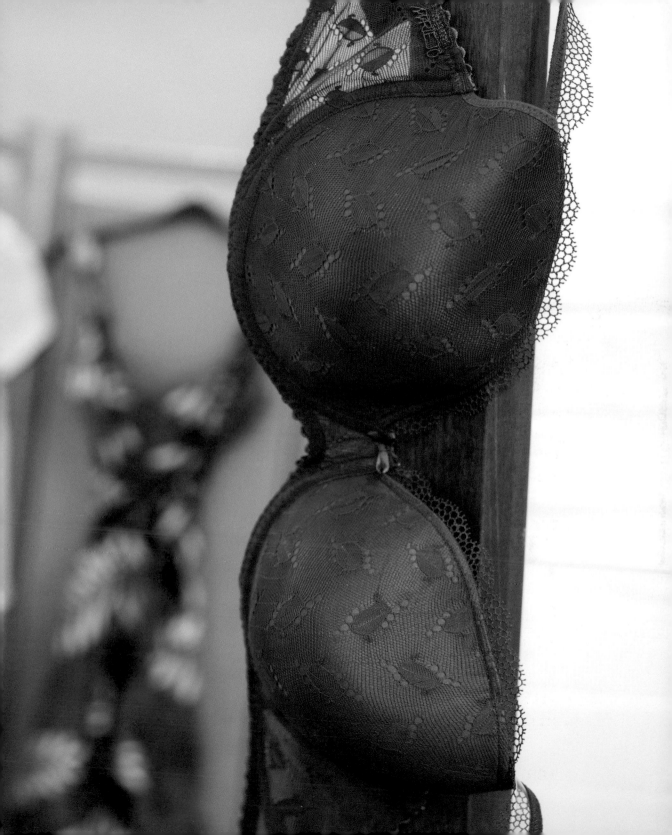

Boobilicious
get that rack out, girl!

Bra sizing

June Kenton, *How to Look Good Naked*'s First Lady of lingerie, thinks that 80 per cent of the women she fits at Rigby and Peller are wearing the wrong size bra. (Go on, admit it; that doesn't even surprise you, does it?) One of the things I've learned from June is that it's so important to have your bra fitted by a trained fitter. Many stores offer this free service, and when you see the difference the right size underwear makes, you will be amazed (I am every week on the show).

I know you know this, but I'm going to say it anyway: it's impossible to guess your bra size. The size and shape of your boobs can change because of diet, sport, pregnancy, even taking certain types of medicine or contraception. You should be measured every six months, and bras that you wear regularly should really be thrown out every year, because they lose their shape and support.

Now here's the shocker. Forget about 'finding out your bra size'. The most important thing is that your bra fits you perfectly, not that it's the same size as all the other bras in your drawer. The shape and therefore the fit of bras can vary enormously between different brands, and even the same style in the same size can be a different fit when it's produced in other fabrics!

So the fit is the most important thing. Which is why bra experts like my lovely June don't even bother using tape measures. Every woman's body shape is different, and those lumps and bumps all need to be taken into account.

The only way to find your correct fit is to keep trying bras until you find the one that is perfect for you. I really would recommend you get yourself professionally fitted. But here are some guidelines to help you out.

How to try on a bra

Slip the straps over your shoulders and lower your breasts into the cups. Bend over from the waist, then fasten the band around your back. When you stand up, you can adjust the fit for comfort.

The hooks

Always wear the bra on the loosest fitting when it's new. The tighter clasps are for when the bra loosens over time (anything up to a few inches!) because of washing and wearing.

The band

The most support from the bra actually comes from the band around your ribs, not the straps or the cups. You should be able to run a finger underneath the band. If you can't, it's too tight. If you can fit more than one finger underneath, it's too loose.

The band should sit in the smallest part of your back (adjust the shoulder straps as needed). It should be horizontal: level front and back. If it's riding up your back, it's probably too big, so try a smaller band size.

The cups

Your boobs should sit right in the cup, with no overspill. Don't think that overspill is a good way to make your rack look bigger: that's what padded and push-ups bras are for, and even with those your boobs should still sit in the cup. If the cups are digging in to create a double boob effect (don't be greedy!), try a larger cup size.

If moulded cups are loose (or you have a gap at your armpit) or if your unpadded bra cups are baggy, go down a cup size. But if there is creasing just around the nipple, you need a smaller band size, to pull the bra back onto your boobs.

The under-wiring

Under-wiring should curve around your hooters, but never dig into them. If it does, you need to go up a cup size. Push on the wire to see if it has any 'give'; if it does, it's sitting on your boobs, not on your rib cage and you need a bigger cup size. If your boobs are falling out of the bottom of the under-wire you need a smaller band size and a bigger cup size.

The centre panel

The centre panel should sit flat against your breastbone, but you should be able to slide a finger underneath. If it's loose, go up a cup size. If it's too tight, you should go up a band size.

The shoulder straps

If the shoulder straps are digging in, or leaving red marks, try loosening them. If this doesn't work, your band is probably too big: it should be supporting your boobs, not the shoulder straps. So try going down a band size. If the straps keep falling off your shoulders, simply tighten them up. A well-fitted bra will still give you support, even when you slip off the shoulder straps.

The final tests

Your bra should lift your chest to just the right height. Bend one arm at the elbow to form a right angle, then lay your arm across your middle. Your bust should be halfway between your shoulder and elbow.

Your bra should not ride up when you lift your arms in the air. Move around in your bra to check that it doesn't pinch or rub when you move.

Try on a tight Lycra T-shirt to check for fleshy lumps and bumps around the bra.

YOUR LINGERIE WARDROBE
- Everyone should have two different types of underwear. Everyday (but pretty) underwear, and magic underwear. The magic underwear should be under lock and key. No one ever need know about that but you...

The Best Lingerie for your Body Shape

Juicy Girl ...

pear shaped but oh so juicy

Pretty

This boob-bolstering in-your-face bra will make your hooters look as big as possible. This is a push-up, plunge style and totally changes her proportions. It's all eyes on the cleavage! The pants are brief with a high-cut, thigh-slimming leg, but still have enough support to boost the bottom.

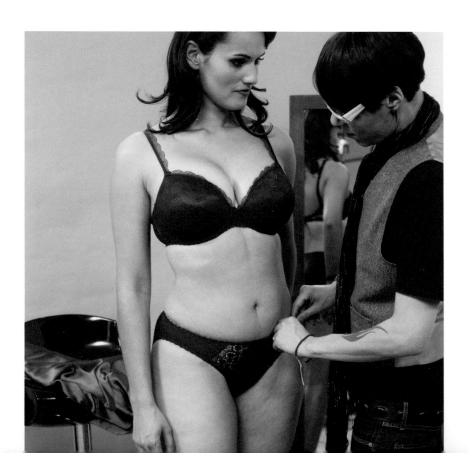

Magic

As support underwear goes, this is some of the prettiest I've ever seen, so if you do let your fella see you in them, you've got maybe a 10 per cent chance of him not running out of the door in terror! Plus the lace edging won't dig into fuller thighs. For pears, it's all about major control around the hips: these cycling shorts really hold everything in and smooth out your silhouette. For pear shapes the strict rule of thumb is always to have a supportive bra to boost your rack, so you balance that silhouette.

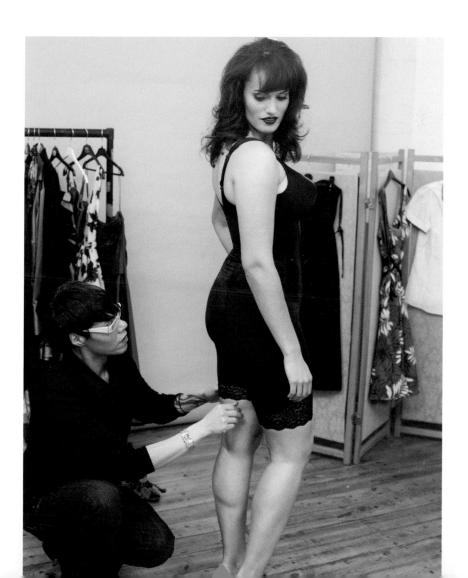

Swimwear

I chose an eye-foxing patterned bikini and added a necklace to bring the focus up towards her gorgeous face. The pattern will make your boobs look bigger, and the briefs are a small plain-cut boy short, taking the attention from Southampton to Manchester, if you know what I mean! The supportive padded style with wide straps gives the upper body a boost.

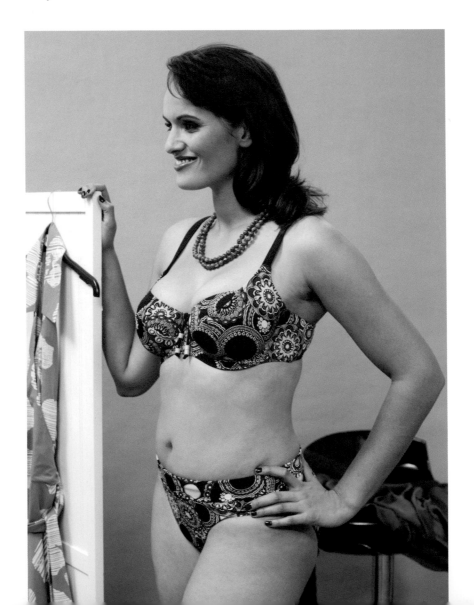

Booty Babe ...

big butt beautiful

Pretty

These are a great cut of panties. It's all in the low-cut leg; they sit underneath the bum, so they offer support, but the leg holes are nicely angled so they're still very flattering on the thighs, and don't cut in. Fuller briefs are much more flattering than, say, a string thong on a juicy booty.

The bra has wide straps that broaden the upper body to even out your curves, and it's a plunge cut for more boob: pushing them up puts some of the attention on that sexy rack of yours instead of your ass.

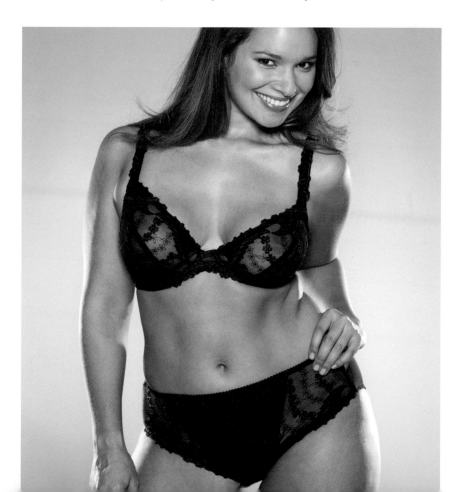

Magic

These are support shorts; they're like cycling shorts, only with double the control elastic on the bum, so you've got extra support in the rear. It's important to remember that support shorts won't dramatically minimise your bottom (which would be a crime!), but it will smooth out any lumps to give you a smoother finish. A full-on boob-boosting bra will even out your silhouette front and back.

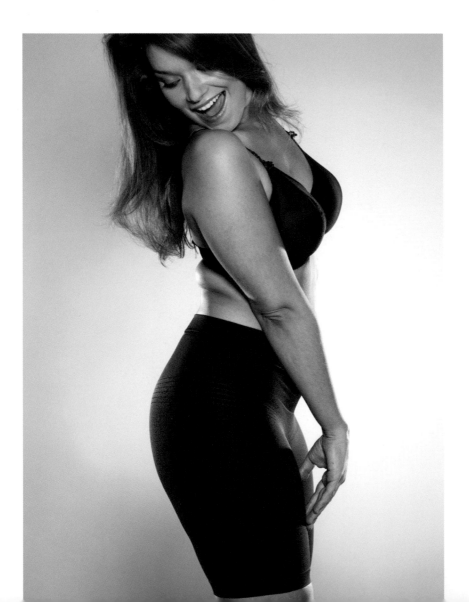

Swimwear

The vertical stripe is obviously a great way of lengthening your body. And if you're still self-conscious, a sarong is the easiest way to cover up but still look sexy. A big detail like this flower motif to one side does no harm: it cuts into your waist, giving an hourglass shape. The built-in bra boosts your cleavage even more (just because you're in a swimsuit instead of a bikini doesn't mean you can't have boobilicious appeal). The low-cut legs mean the suit can offer good support to the bottom. Just be careful not to get water-logged in low-cut suits: you don't want to end up with a bum-full of ocean!

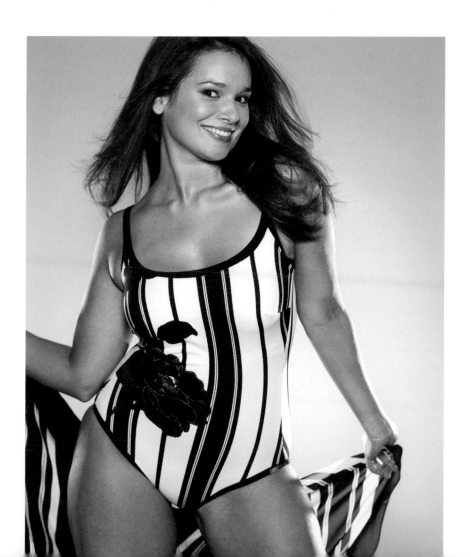

Petite Girl ...

small but perfectly formed

Pretty

This half-cup padded plunge bra will boost your boobs. The angled cups make them look larger, and draw attention to your cleavage. The lighter colour and pattern of the white lace will also make you look bigger and curvier; plus the fabric is slightly see-through, which is a little bit risqué ... The high-thigh-cut panty extends your legs, and that vertical line on the briefs elongates the lower body.

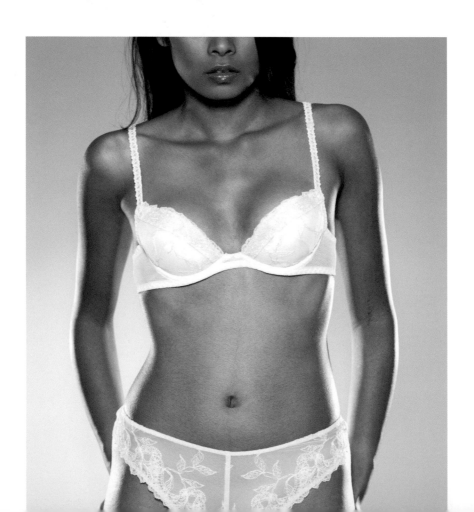

Magic

Again, this is the classic half-cup padded plunge bra, which is best for maximizing your boobs. Deep pants add curves to your hips, and even in slimming black give you a more substantial visual presence. A low-slung brief with high-cut legs will lengthen your pins.

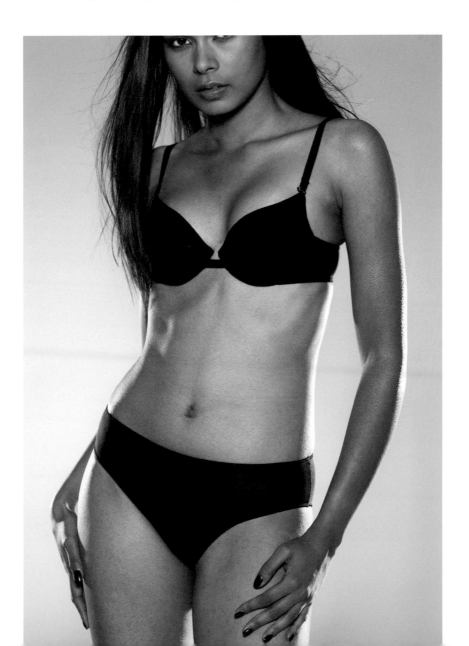

Swimwear

Only if you're petite can you can get away with the triangle string bikini. The patterned fabric gives your chest and bottom more depth and curves; small, subtle prints like this are better for your frame. The deep V neckline formed by the triangular cups give the illusion of cleavage, taking the focus from your neck down to your chest. The string ties on the side of the low-slung briefs break up the line of your body, adding subtle width to the hips.

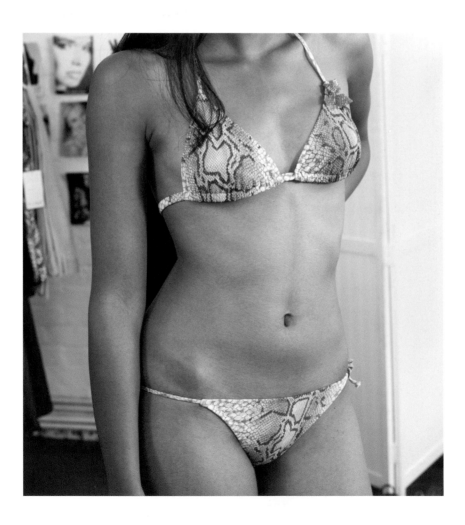

Sexy Broad ...

no curves but who cares

Pretty

This pretty daily underwear has light boning in it that helps to give you the curves you're always after. It's also incredibly sexy! I've chosen a microfibre brief for a seamless look, but the mesh panels keep it feminine and pretty.

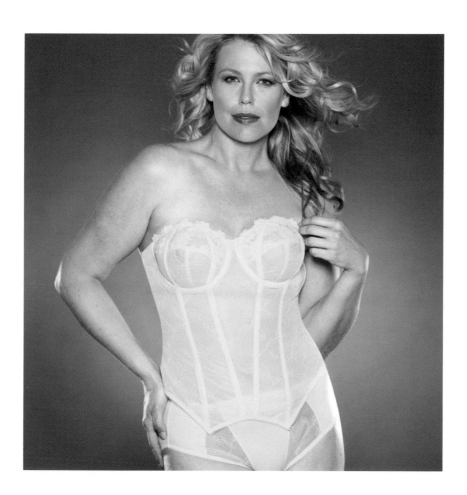

Magic

Look at the waist on that! This foxy satin corset gives you curves and looks seriously sophisticated too. The sweetheart-shaped cups boost the boobs, the corset draws in the waist, and the boy shorts give coverage and emphasize the bottom, so that you go from no curves to hourglass! The vertical line of the fastenings also elongate the line of the body. And you're Lady Marmalade...

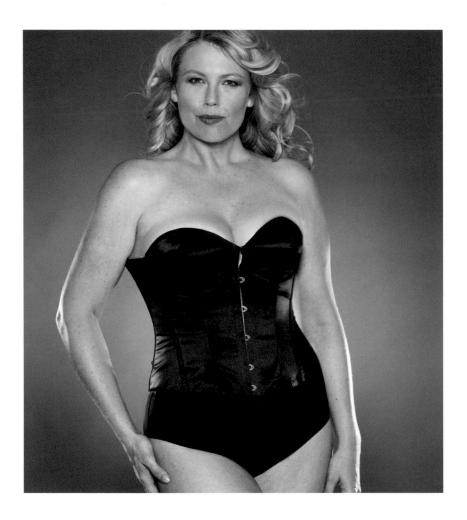

Swimwear

If you've got no curves, this is liposuction in a garment. There is so much support and control-panelling in this swimsuit, that I have to warn you, if you do get it on, don't expect to get it off again. But it is amazing, because there's no flesh spilling out, so where does it go?

This style is very flattering too, though, because black is very slimming. Also, a strapless style will make you appear more curvaceous by emphasizing the arms, and making the shoulders look broader.

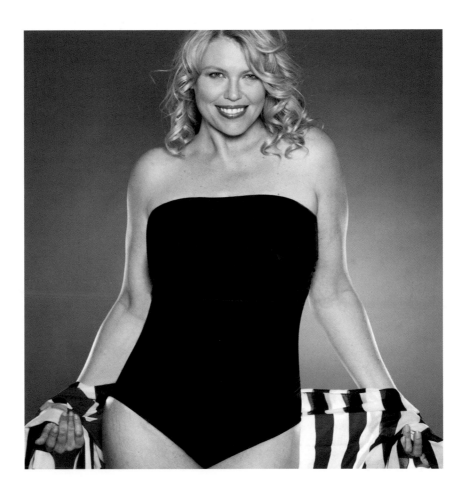

Curvy Girl ...

hourglass is the new black

Pretty

This is a proper full-cup balcony bra, to boost your boobs up around your neck! With an hourglass silhouette, the first thing you need is good support; so this is a super-structured scaffold bra, but it's still gorgeous. This style will give you fantastic support and make your boobs appear broader and bigger – and that tiny waist of yours even smaller. The wide straps have pretty detailing, but are strong enough to support you.

These are perfect pants! They're substantial enough for supporting your bottom, plus all that fabric makes the waist look smaller in between.

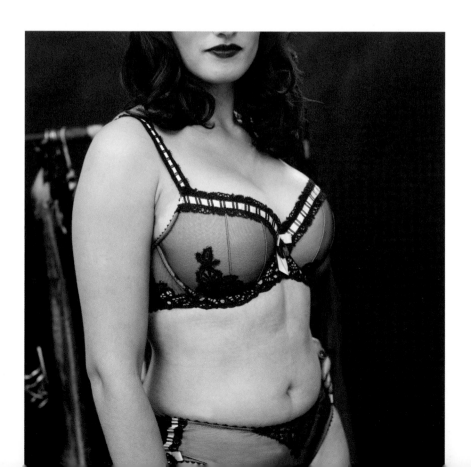

Magic

As we know, basque is the new black. There is nothing more beautiful than an hourglass figure in old-fashioned lingerie! The lacing up the back is mainly for aesthetic value, but it does mean you have a cleaner finish on the front. It brings your waist in, making it look even tinier. And again, the big pants offer support, and look right with the major statement of the basque.

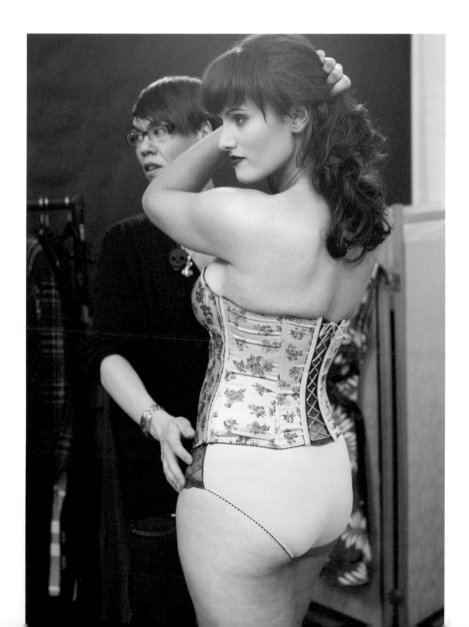

Swimwear

This swimsuit is perfectly made for an hourglass figure! It is constructed of panels, so that it is actually cut in a shape that's fitted to flatter the body, instead of just relying on Lycra to hold everything in. The belt is low-slung, so that it emphasizes the hips, making the waist look smaller. The halter-neck also boosts your rack. By highlighting your boobs and bottom, it emphasizes your tiny waist, accentuating your to-die-for hourglass silhouette.

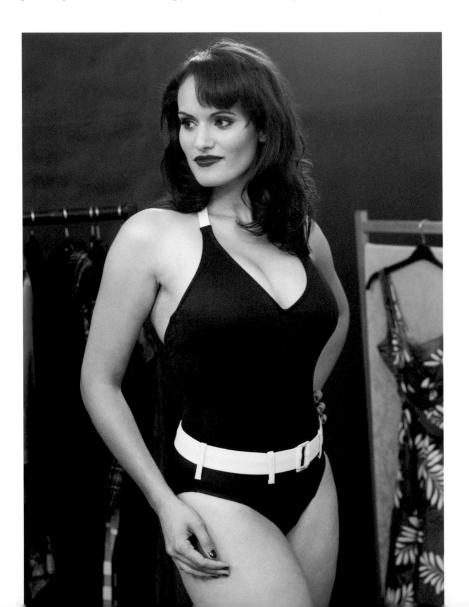

Bellyssimo Babe ...

paunchy but raunchy

Pretty

The balcony bra is great for women with a big stomach; it's all about pushing your rack out in front, to lessen the depth of the belly.

   The high-cut knicker has a waistband that sits on the belly: too low and
you'd get a muffin top; too high, and it will just emphasize the curve of the
belly. The waistband is in relaxed elastic, so that it clings but doesn't dig in
tightly. For those with weight on the hips and legs as well, the lace finish on
the bottom of the briefs is great because it doesn't cut in like elastic would.

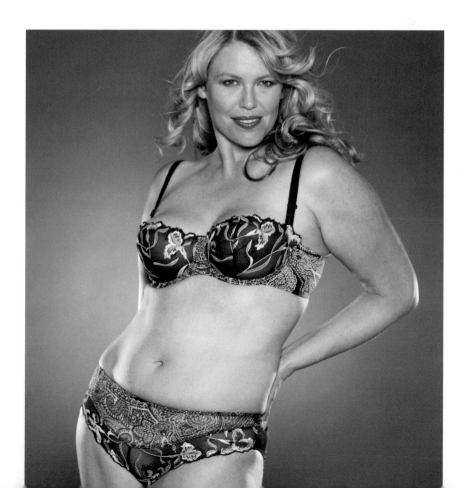

Magic

Obviously we call these knickers apple-catchers – they practically come up to your neck! These miracle pants hold in your entire stomach with a strong panel of elastic. Our model had great thighs, but you could wear the shorts version if you wanted to minimize that area too. We've got a very supportive bra to boost your boobs up and forwards, so that they have more depth than the stomach. I actually think this is quite a flattering set of support underwear for anyone with a big stomach, because the two pieces are so substantial, in that 1950s style, that the midsection looks much less prominent in comparison.

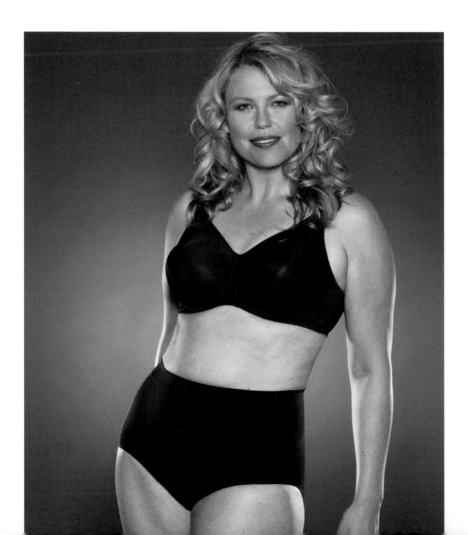

Swimwear

This is the perfect swimwear for someone with a big belly, because it looks like separates, but it's actually an all-in-one, so you don't get any bulk where the pieces come together. This swimsuit contains about 6 million per cent Lycra too, so it really smoothes out your silhouette, flattening the stomach. It's low-cut on the hips, so it's supportive around your bottom. It's also a great built-in bra, very supportive, so it's almost like a miracle-underwear suit.

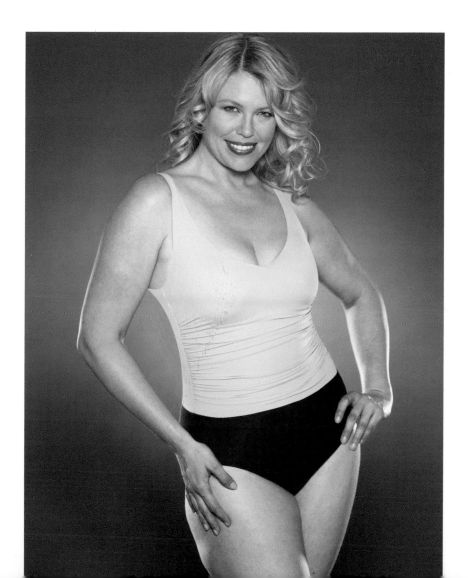

Cleavage Diva …

top heavy and traffic stopping

Pretty

Sometimes if you're top-heavy you want to really go for it, lingerie-wise. And sometimes you don't. If you want to play your fantastic rack down a little, a sexy négligé is a great way to slim and lengthen your silhouette, plus it will hide your boobs without covering them up. The bra is just a gorgeous, supportive, full-cup bra with cheeky half-cup detailing. And again, sheer sexy pants are full-on enough to balance your silhouette.

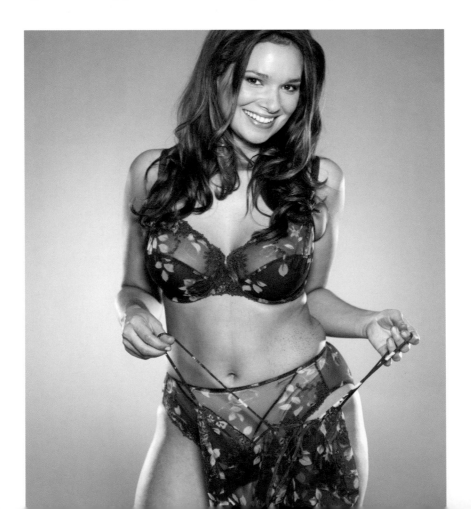

Magic

This support bra is not dissimilar to a sports bra – just a bit sexier! It is very supportive and pushes your rack up, up, up. It's great for dividing your boobs, to avoid ending up with the dreaded mono-boob shelf! Also, the deep V-neck means you can still wear your oh-so-flattering low vertical neckline.

For top-heavy ladies, the trick is to find sexy but substantial pants. These smooth out any lumps and the low-cut lace legs emphasize your bottom without cutting into your thighs.

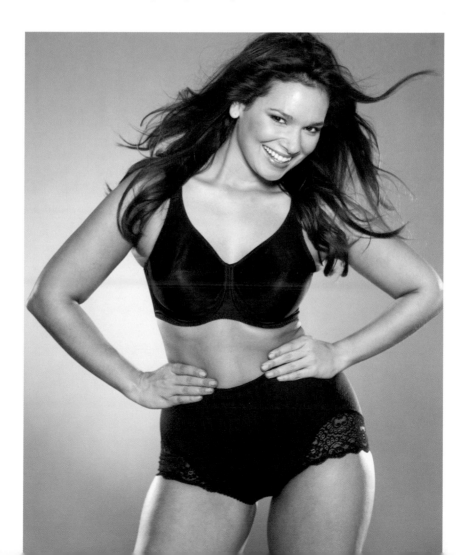

Swimwear

This swimsuit is a minimizing style. It spreads your rack out width-wise, to stop you looking too top-heavy. This is better than a style that just flattens you down, which can be really unflattering. It also pushes your boobs away from each other, which makes them appear smaller. Underwired cups and wide-apart straps are great for support.

The substantial briefs are great for emphasizing your derrière, and balancing out your boobs.

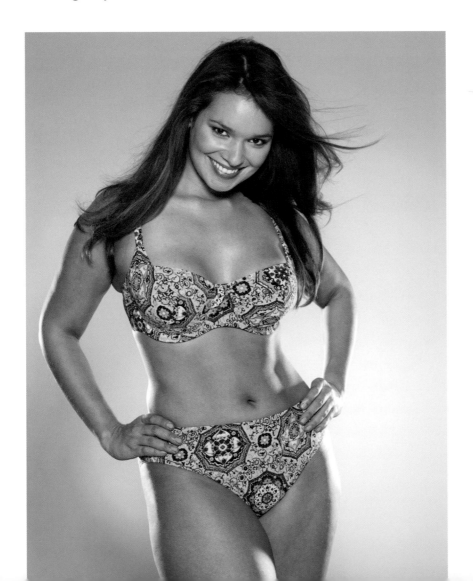

Slim and Sexy ...

skinny and fabulous

Pretty

If you're not quite an A-cup, a push-up padded plunge bra pulls out all the tricks to help you make mountains out of molehills. The diagonal cut of the cups will make you appear curvier. The high-legged thong lengthens the leg, and the sides are wide enough to put emphasis on the hips. A light-coloured patterned fabric like white lace will also give you a greater physical presence and emphasize your boobs and hips, making you look more curvaceous.

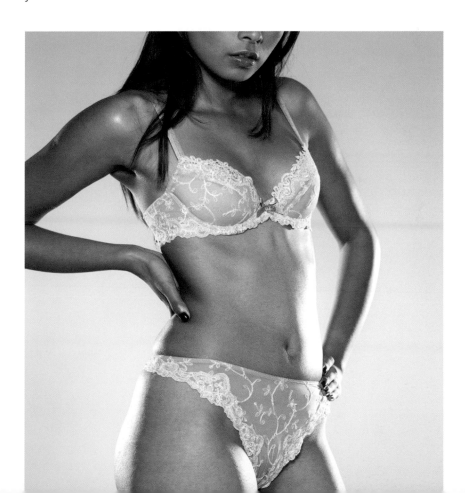

Magic

If you're flat-chested, you need chicken fillets. Cheap, simple and so much less painful than surgery, these are waiflike celebrities' favourite secret weapon. They're even handbag-sized so you can whip 'em out before your partner sees them! They also come in different cup sizes, so you can adjust your breasts, bigger or smaller according to your mood (which makes top-heavy women very jealous). Plus you can move them around to create different effects: wide and forward for the 1950s sweater-girl style, or close together and up for the Girls Aloud cleavage. An inch to the left or right and you shift decades.

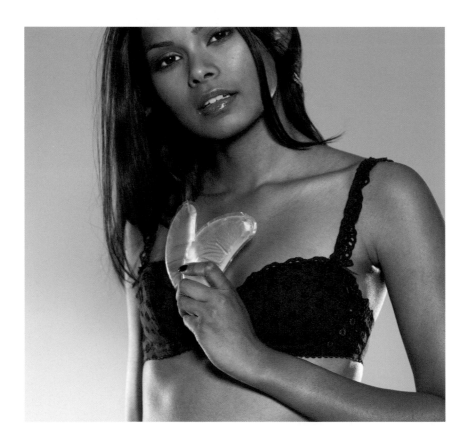

Swimwear

Horizontal stripes are your best friend! They will broaden your silhouette at the breasts and hips. This halter-neck string style will point down to your cleavage, making your boobs appear bigger either side. This kind of elaborate top will draw more attention to your chest.

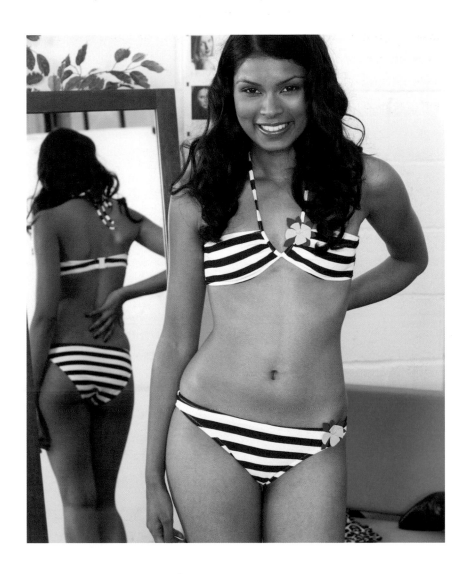

Gok's Golden Rules

- Never wear your underwear tighter than it needs to be. I hate visible panty lines and that pigskin-drum effect from too-tight supportwear.

- If you're wearing anything bigger than a B cup, you definitely need under-wiring.

- Invest as much time, effort and money into buying underwear as you do in your visible wardrobe; never let your underwear become an afterthought.

- Buy chicken fillets and nipple flowers (sticky pads that cover up pokey nipples) now! You never know when an outfit will need them.

- If you take exercise without wearing a sports bra, you will get stretch marks that nothing other than surgery can get rid off.

- Sometimes lingerie can be an inspiration for a whole outfit. I might style an outfit starting with the lace on a bra, or some control pants might make me want to come up with an outfit to showcase the bum because it looks so good.

- Underwear is as much an expression of your personality as your hair or your shoes. Let your partner know you're feeling sexy by wearing something lacy. Let your lingerie do the talking (and let his fingers do the walking). Ding dong...

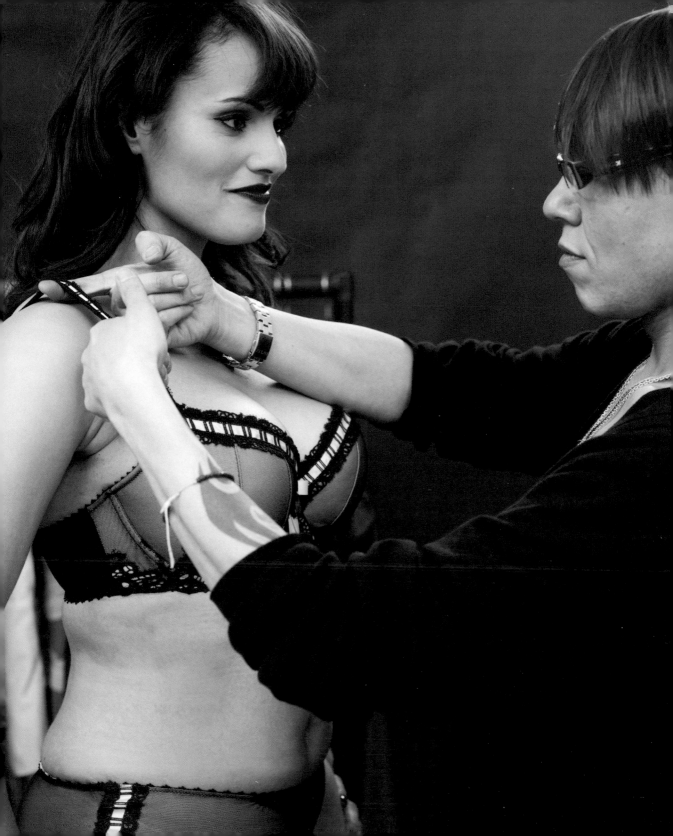

Body Scrumptious…

beauty tips for fashion foxes

This chapter is all about you, foxy lady, and no one else – taking care of yourself, pampering yourself and appreciating yourself. Image and style aren't just about the clothes you wear – they're about still being fabulous when the clothes come off. And make no mistake, you are fabulous!

To me, style is just as much about how you feel, how you hold yourself, the touch of your skin and the smell of your hair, as the cut of a classic YSL tuxedo. Because, my gorgeous, what's the point of spending good money on beautiful clothes, if when you take them off you don't like what you see? So we're going to focus on your body, inside and out, and look at those crafty adjustments and fast fixes that can make a dramatic difference – let's call them Gok's Tricks of the Trade…

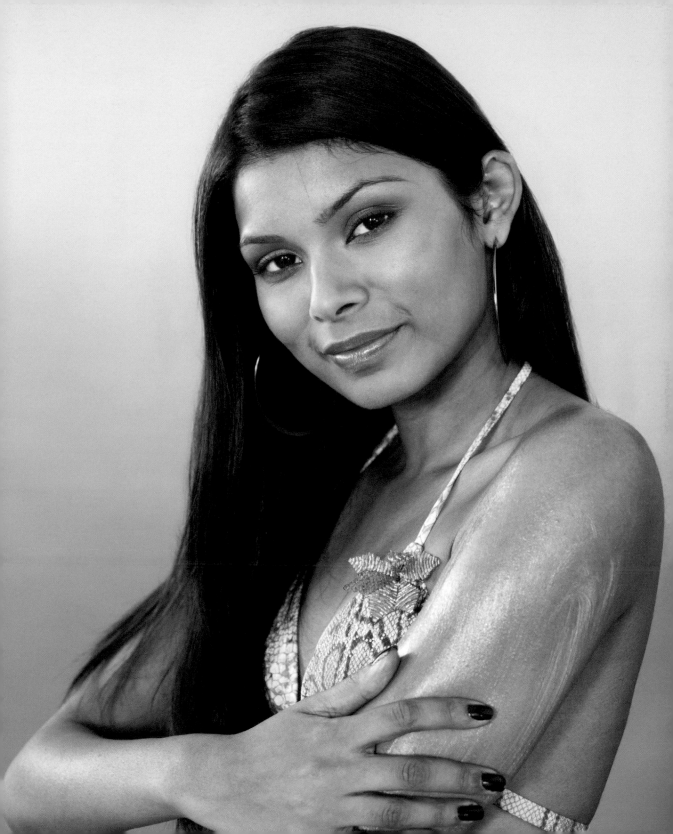

The Naked Truth: Assessment

Bodies come in all different shapes and sizes. And I know from my show that the moment you start realizing this, your life will be improved ten-fold.

The Line-up

If *How to Look Good Naked* taught me one thing, it's that many women have an overly negative image of how they look. This is why we do the line-up on the programme – where women have to assess how big they think their bottom/boobs/tummy are, compared to those of a row of strangers.

Without fail, each of the women always gets it wrong. And none of them ever *under*estimates their body size. Just as revealingly, they all underestimate the sizes of the other women in the line-up. This is a good lesson to learn: other people see you as skinnier than you actually are (yay!). But it also tells us that we are a lot harder on ourselves than we are on other people. And this, my pretty, has got to stop.

Positive Feedback

I love the 'reveal' part of the show, where we see each woman, newly made-over and in a gorgeous outfit. But the real breakthrough for all the women on the show is understanding that they have got the state of their bodies totally out of perspective.

This is helped by me naughtily projecting their naked bodies onto buildings, then asking for feedback from members of the public – or even people they know. The feedback is always really positive (and unprompted!) and often, the woman's most hated body part turns out to be the part that gets the most compliments.

OK, not everybody can appear on my show, but you can still get that positive feedback – and where better to start than with your nearest and dearest. I want you to ask three people, maybe a friend, a sister, a partner, what your best bits are. It's always a fun conversation and, of course, a total ego trip and you can then do the same for them in return. Some of the answers might be really obvious (if you've got, say, a great rack, or amazing eyes). But you will probably be surprised by some of the other parts they mention, because we don't always notice our best assets.

And with that confidence boost, you're ready for the next step, sexy lady. (No, I'm not going to ask you to get all your friends to line up in their underwear; although if you do, I'd love to know how it goes!)

Be your own best friend – not your own worst critic!

The Mirror Moment

I want you to take a look at your body in the mirror as we do in the show. I mean really look at yourself, honey. If it's been a while (and you even need to go out and buy a full-length mirror first!), then be brave – it's the first step to making a difference to how you feel about yourself and see yourself. You're not alone, you'd be surprised how body-unconfident some of the world's most beautiful women are.

Now look at your bod. Of course, the first things you are going to notice are the bits you like least. Believe me, everyone has parts of their body they don't like (or they don't like any more), including me; I really hate my double chin (no, don't start looking for it in all the photos!).

So here's the deal. For every negative thought you have about a body part, you have to say something positive, for balance. Acknowledge the bits that you don't love, and focus on the bits you do. These are the parts we're going to dress up!

To get started, I'm going to give you three New You resolutions:

1. Stop Being Negative

Don't be so hard on yourself, girl. This is really important. Stop thinking negative things and only ever let yourself think positive things about your body, because you will start to believe them.

Hand in hand with this, stop being negative or envious about other people's bodies; taking a 'them and us' attitude to beauty is self-fulfilling. Learn the art of acceptance, for yourself and others.

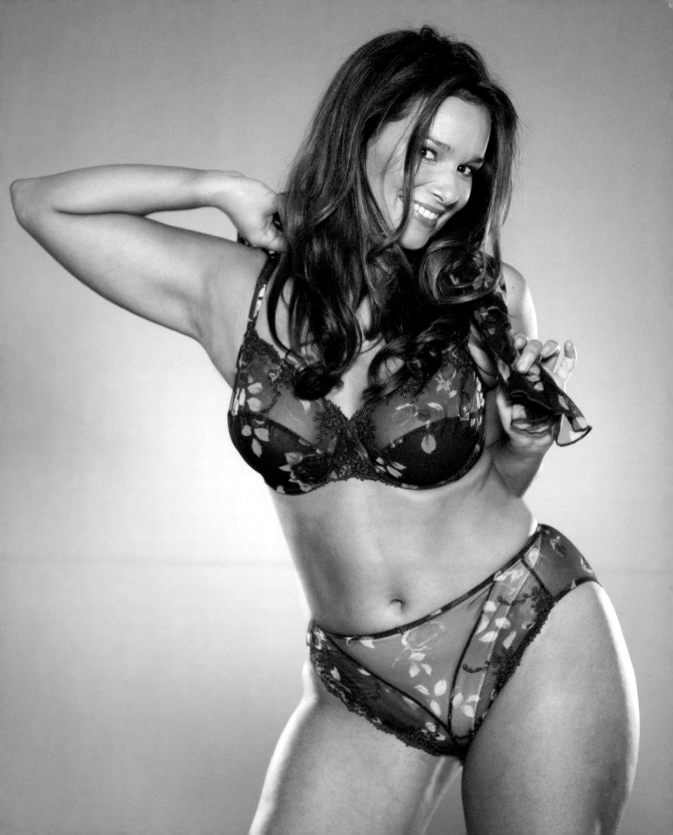

2. Keep an Overall Perspective

Now that you've completed the mirror exercise, I want you to stop seeing your body in different parts – good parts and bad parts. We tend to be so busy focusing on the body parts we hate, that we never get round to noticing the beautiful parts we love, and, just as importantly, getting the overall picture, which is rarely as bad as we think. So from now on, I want you to stand back, and only ever think of your body as a whole beautiful image.

3. Fake It 'til You Make It

I'll let you into a little secret: confidence and contentment are as attractive as beauty. We can all think of women who aren't traditionally beautiful, but who just have something about them. This aura is nearly always self-confidence. And it is devastatingly attractive.

Self-confidence is there for the taking – you just have to decide to have it, honey. Believing you are self-confident will certainly convince other people, and eventually, yourself.

A great way to fake self-confidence is great posture. Carrying yourself with confidence will convince everyone that you're proud of your body. So shoulders back, chin up, walk as tall as you can, sweet lips. Of course, this new attitude won't happen overnight. Like any great relationship, the one between you and your body is going to take time.

Naked Body: Your Skin

The best thing you can do for your body is care for your skin.

Moisturize

Moisturizing is a daily pleasure every girl needs and that includes you. Yes, it nourishes the skin, keeping it soft and supple, and yes, it gets the circulation going, improving skin tone. But more than that, it's your chance to relax and get to know and love your body.

And remember, touch, not sight, is our most heightened sense. So the next time you're stripping off in front of 'him indoors' and busy worrying about how your love handles look, all he's thinking about is how amazingly soft your skin feels ... And you can complete the sensual experience by layering fragrance with a matching shower gel, moisturizer and perfume to create a longer lasting scent.

Exfoliate

The other way to keep your skin super-soft is to exfoliate. It's an easy treatment to do in the shower in the mornings and a good scrubbing will do more than just remove all your dead skin cells – it will really wake you up and invigorate you. To get the blood flowing around your skin and for that gorgeous goddess glow, make sure you rub in a circular motion up towards your heart. You'll notice the difference and your skin will feel so much softer afterwards. Salt scrubs are great body exfoliators – I make my own version at home with olive oil and coarse salt grains.

Exfoliation is also a great way to prepare the skin for other products like body lotion or fake tan, which work better on smooth, clean skin. So get exfoliating, foxy lady.

Sun Protection

I think everyone knows about the dangers of lying in the sun now. Tanning is the no. 1 cause of skin cancer, as well as the no. 1 cause of skin ageing and wrinkles. Fortunately, self-tanning products are so effective and easy to use now, there's no need to exposure your skin to harmful rays.

I use a self-tanning body lotion because I'm so pasty, and I have to look healthy and groomed for my work. I feel like it just gives me a bit of a lift.

Over the years, I've tested a lot of fake tanning products, both on myself and models, and I find that the daily gradual self-tanning products are far better than the spray tans or the instant colour tans, which often go streaky or too dark (or make you smell like bacon!).

Best of all, try to find a self-tanning product that also contains sun protection.

Celebrity Glow

That special glow celebrities have ... is it star quality? Inner beauty? Fame? No, girlfriend, it's iridescent body lotion.

This is every celebrity's essential body product. I swear by it on shoots. It gives a sheen to your skin, which highlights the muscles (I swear it makes your limbs look slimmer) and reflects the light in an incredibly soft, flattering way, giving you the most amazing glow.

You will never see any bare celebrity flesh without this product on it, whether on a shoot or the red carpet. Get yourself a bottle and you'll see why.

Gok's Golden Rules for Skin

- Nourish your skin and face with moisturizing body lotions and face masks.

- Always protect your face with a daily moisturizer containing at least SPF 15.

- Keep your skin glowing with self-tanning products and iridescent lotions.

- Exfoliate your skin to keep it soft – salt scrubs for the body, and AHAs for the face. Silky smooth skin drives fellas wild!

- Drink more water to improve your complexion.

Naked Face: Your Complexion

I know you've heard it before, honey, but it really is important to drink enough water. Water flushes out toxins from your system, and plumps up the skin to help diminish fine lines. Most people's skin is dehydrated, even if we don't realize it. Often when people think they're hungry, they're actually thirsty, so they end up eating when their body is really craving a glass of water.

And if you're still doubting that water can make any difference to your skin ... let me put it this way: as a make up artist, I can always tell from a client's face whether they had been a) drinking lots of water and b) moisturizing. So make sure you have a 2-litre bottle of water by your side each day and get drinking (not all at once!). And don't worry about peeing all day long, your system will get back to normal after the first couple of days.

Hands Off

Try to avoid touching your face as much as you can. Even clean hands are covered in oil, dirt, and bacteria, which can be transferred to your skin, causing spots. Another tip is to launder your pillowcase at least once a week. It's kind of obvious, but pressing your face against dirty fabric every night is not good for the complexion.

Pore Cleansing Strips

Obviously, we all get bad breakouts once in a while. But squeezing your spots, blackheads and blemishes really damages your skin. I am a big fan of those rip-off pore cleansing strips; they totally clean your skin out. If you're a squeezer, I can't recommend them highly enough.

Face Masks

I'm a huge fan of face masks – they only take ten minutes to work their magic and are the beauty equivalent of a Do Not Disturb sign. Most people need two masks; one to moisturize (unless your skin is unusually oily), and an AHA mask. AHAs are alpha hydroxy acids, which gently but deeply exfoliate your skin without scrubbing with a gritty cleanser. Regular exfoliation will help combat a dull complexion. AHAs are kinder and more effective than traditional exfoliators. So treat yourself, hot stuff, and try to use the AHA mask followed by the moisturizing mask once a week.

SPF Moisturizer

After cleansing, the daily application of a moisturizer with at least SPF 15 is the most important thing you can do for your face. Whether you've been good or bad in the sun up to now, it is never too late to start taking positive action and protecting your skin from the sun every day.

Home Treatments

I also believe in easy natural remedies. You can never totally understand all the ingredients listed in the products you buy, but homemade treatments are pure, easy, cheap and can be really fun and satisfying to do by yourself or with friends (make a girlie evening of it!).My favourite is mashing up some fresh avocado to apply to my face. It works brilliantly as a moisturizer. Sometimes when I get stressed, I find I get quite bad dry patches on my skin, and this treatment always sorts them out.

Hair

Your no. 1 accessory is your hair, my gorgeous! More than anything else, I really believe your hair can make or break your look (yup; more than make up, even more than fashion).

We all hate bad hair days, and a bad haircut can ruin your life for months. But a great hairstyle will knock years off you, and give you a major confidence boost. For this reason, I recommend you spend as much on your hair as you possibly can. And go for regular haircuts; at least every six weeks.

Style and Condition

This might surprise you, but as far as I'm concerned, style outweighs condition. Of course, blow-drying your style will damage your hair, but what's the alternative? Very few people can carry off wash-and-wear hair. My most important hair tip: never let your hairdresser blow-dry your hair! You'll never be able to copy it yourself when you get home. Instead, get them to teach you how to do it.

To minimize damage; try to keep your dryer on as low a heat setting as possible; slick through some serum and you'll be fine. Changing your parting is a good idea too; you will reveal new shiny undamaged hair. If all that fails, go for regular vegetable-based glossing rinses; it's like a semi-permanent varnish for your hair.

More than anything you can improve the condition of your hair by what you eat. Fish contains omega 3 and essential fatty acids, which are vital for healthy skin, hair and nails. So eat as much as you can and watch your skin, hair and nails turn shiny, shiny, shiny! I promise, you will be amazed.

Home Treatments

Again, I like a good home remedy for hair. I apply freshly-squeezed lemon juice to my hair for shine (be so, so, careful not to get it in your eyes, or any cuts!). Leave it on for ten minutes, then rinse out – it's brilliant. It works by taking away any residue that has built up from hair products. It's also great to use before a deep conditioning treatment.

I used to have longer hair (yes, alright), and when it got in really bad condition I'd rub through some pure sunflower oil and wrap my head in a towel for ten minutes. It really reconditions your hair. And I swear it's just as good as a £50 salon treatment, (seriously, I've tried both). This is great to do at the same time as a face pack, for real pampering.

Gok's Golden Rules for Hair

- Never use leave-in conditioners. These will make your hair look greasy, rather than shiny. Avoid shampoos with built-in conditioners – in my experience they don't do either job well.

- Always get a professional to colour your hair, even if it means going to a salon's model night to get it done for free by a trainee colourist.

- Know how to style your own hair; get your hairdresser to teach you.

- Eat lots of fish; it will make all the difference to your skin, hair and nails.

- Don't keep touching your hair; it'll just make it greasy.

Make up

I love make up. Working as a make up artist on shoots was a dream come true for me. It was my first job in fashion, and I loved that make up could have magical transforming properties. But make up isn't about painting on a new face, it's about enhancing different aspects of your own natural beauty (much more exciting!).

There are two aspects to make up; application and products. In both cases, less is more.

Gok's Big Beauty Clearout

I urge you, girlfriend, to go and get your make up bag now. Don't be shy. Tip it on the table and be honest with yourself. What do you see?

I believe in beauty feng shui: clean out the old to bring in the new. The strict rule of thumb is that if a beauty or make up product has been sitting around unused for three months, give it away or chuck it out. If you're not using it, it's probably for a good reason. And no product is 'too posh' – I'm putting my foot down and insisting you start using it today. Beauty products have an expiry date (and so do people; you might get hit by a bus tomorrow, and that nearly-full pot of deluxe body moisturizer will have been wasted!). Try limiting yourself to just a top ten of products that you use all the time (at least once a month).

How to Avoid: too thick foundation

Most foundations are too thick on their own, so make up artists tend to mix liquid foundation with moisturizer before applying it. This gives a nice lightweight sheer cover and a smooth consistent finish.

Be smart, honey: if you're mixing your foundation with a moisturizer with sun protection, you're doing three steps in one: moisturizer, sun protection and foundation. Brilliant. Your skin tone will vary according to the time of year, so I recommend getting a consultant to test the colour on your skin *every time you buy a new foundation*. Besides, you'll never find out if another product suits you better.

How to Avoid: chalky concealer

Go carefully, girl, if your concealer is too light, it's only gonna draw more attention to those dark circles or spots! Choose a slightly yellow shade to counteract the blue tones of under-eye shadows – make sure it's one or two shades lighter than your skin tone. Use as little as you can, and build it up by patting it on with your fingertip. If you suffer from really dark circles, consider using fake tan on your face.

How to Avoid: unnatural blusher or bronzer

Wearing too much blusher or bronzer is as bad as not wearing any at all, my gorgeous. My favourite sneaky tip for a sexy natural blush is to use your lipstick as a blusher too. Dab (not draw) some lipstick onto the back of your hand, then, with your index finger, dab some gently onto the apples of your cheeks (the chubby bits when you smile). Build up the colour gradually. I love this trick; it blends easily and gives a good colour match.

How to Avoid: spidery lashes

Make up artists hardly ever choose waterproof mascara over the regular kind, as it is always more drying on your lashes and therefore much more likely to make them go spidery. And make sure you replace your mascara every three months. Any longer and the mascara will start to dry out, which makes it go on clumpy.

Make up artists like to wiggle the wand at the base of the lashes, as it's the mascara at the roots, not the tips, that makes your lashes look longer. My favourite method is to apply mascara to the back of your lashes first, really layering it on and applying second or third coats immediately (waiting for each coat to dry between applications is what makes the lashes clump). Then immediately give one steady sweep from the roots to the tips of the front of your lashes. *Et voilà* – long, full lashes!

Keep Updating Your Make up

Make up styles change, just as fashion does; you wouldn't be seen dead in culottes or crushed velvet now, would you? But you might still be wearing the same make up you wore ten years ago. Don't get stuck in a time warp. Because, honey, sure as anything, your face hasn't...

Besides, it's so much fun to try new styles. Don't be afraid to experiment and try new products. Get a complimentary makeover on a beauty counter (check the assistant's own make up out first, maybe!). Give them free reign and you'll be surprised how many great ideas you pick up.

Gadgets

Don't waste money on beauty gadgets – they're always useless. You'll use them once and then never again. If someone wants to buy you a present, ask for perfume or treatment vouchers instead. The only gadget in my shoot kit is a pair of old-fashioned eyelash curlers.

Gok's Golden Rules for Make up

- New looks are always worth trying; experiment a little, copy looks from magazines or get a free makeover at the beauty counter.

- Always mix your foundation with moisturizer to give better coverage and a sheerer finish.

- Concealer must only be a shade lighter than your foundation.

- Limit your make up products to your top ten essentials.

- Don't overdo your make up when you're feeling tired and hung over; less is more, and focus on the blusher.

How to Look Good Naked...

sneaky tips for cheeky girls

So, foxy lady, you know you look good with your clothes on, but how about taking it one step further and wowing your fella with your clothes off? There's a reason why this book's called *How to Look Good Naked*!

The naked photo-shoot is one of my favourite parts of the show. I love seeing how comfortable my girls have got with their bodies by the end of our time together; comfortable enough to agree to being photographed naked! They all look fantastic. And so will you, you naughty minx!

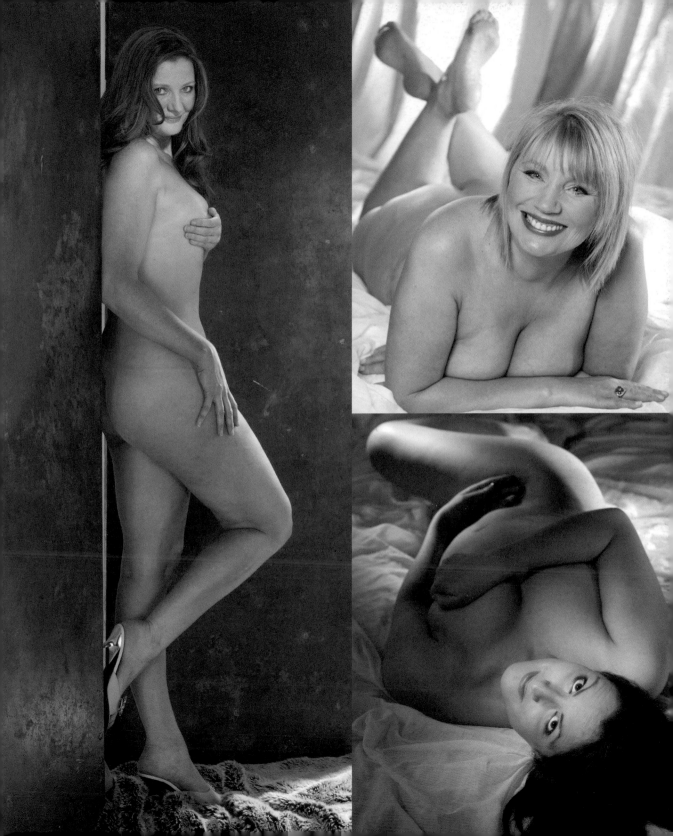

My girls on the show were in safe hands (as it were!). I had worked on celebrity photo-shoots with top photographer Mike Owen for years, so I knew he was the man for the job. Not only does Mike take amazing pictures, with beautiful lighting, he's also great at putting his models at their ease. I can get my girls looking gorgeous, but he's the guy who knows all the best poses, and how to show anyone's best sides. And I think you can really see that in these photos.

Mike and I thought it would be fun to give you some tips on how to do your own naked photo-shoot. After all, if you know how to look good naked, shouldn't you capture it for posterity?

'For a lot of women, a nude portrait is a lovely way to remember yourself and something to be proud of as you get older,' says Mike. Also, it's a lovely thing to do with your partner, and it can be a very special and romantic experience.

So if you ever fancy having a bit of fun with your fella, here are Mike's top tips for your own private photo-shoots. There's nothing like a bit of lights, camera, action to put-back the va-va-voom in the bedroom!

- First of all, invest in a digital camera, so you can edit the pictures as you go along. And, more importantly, you won't have to take your film into a shop to be developed!
- Next, think about where you want to shoot.
- Keep the background simple, shooting against soft colours and/or soft fabrics, which will flatter your skin and will help you remain the central focus. Avoid bright colours or jazzy prints which will be distracting.
- Keeping the room warm will always help to make you more comfortable!
- Don't feel you have to take everything off for a 'nude' portrait. If you don't want to go fully naked, don't worry. It's often sexier to keep parts of you hidden, and leave something to the imagination.

If you love your boobs

Lie on your front, leaning on one bent arm resting in front of your boobs. This will focus all attention on your fabulous rack, while also framing them in a subtle way.

If you're boob-shy

Cross your hands over your chest, holding a boob in each hand, pulling your shoulders slightly back. Push upwards to give a more pert appearance; instant boob lift! Or lie on your back with your arms draped above your head.

If you love your arms

Pose sideways leaning up against a wall, with your arms bent at right angles and your hands clasped. This will make your muscles stand out, and highlight the sexy curves of your arms.

If you're arm-shy

Stand up, holding one arm down to the side, but slightly behind your body. With the other arm, place your hand on your hip and move the arm as far forward as possible.

If you love your waist

If you're a curvy girl, why not pose sitting down with your back to the camera, looking over one shoulder? This will make your curvaceous silhouette the main focus of the picture.

If you're waist-shy

Sit ½ on to the camera. Have one leg bent at the knee and drape your arm along your thigh – this will conceal your middle section.

If you love your tummy

Stand ½ on to the camera, with your hands on your hips. Your fingers will focus attention on your yummy tummy.

If you're tummy-shy

Lie on your stomach! Or lie on your back, which will flatten out your stomach, and drape one arm over your tummy.

If you love your booty

You can create a nicer shape to your bottom by straddling a chair, stretching your legs, and leaning slightly forward. This will make your bootylicious bottom look even more pert.

If you're booty-shy

Lie on your front, leaning up on one bent arm; your head and shoulders will conceal your wayward booty.

If you love your thighs

Pose standing leaning up against a wall, bend one leg, standing on tip toe. This will elongate your thigh and make it the sexy focus of the picture.

If you're thigh-shy

Cross the top of your legs over, to narrow that area, or drape an arm down one thigh to conceal part of it.

If you love your legs

Pose sitting straddling a chair, which will stretch your fabulous legs out in front, and make them appear even more toned.

If you're leg-shy

This might sound obvious; but crop the picture at your hips! Otherwise, it's always more flattering to have one leg slightly further forward. And don't forget your heels!

Best All-round Pose

Lie on your back on a bed, with your head slightly tilted back over the edge of the bed. This is a very good way to stretch your neck, let the weight fall off your face, and highlight your bone structure. Casually drape your hands and arms over any parts of yourself you wish to conceal.

This pose will make you feel like the sexiest woman alive – and you can guarantee that your fella behind the camera will be thinking the same.

Mike's Golden Rules for Nude Portraits

- Never shoot in direct sunlight or harsh artificial light; both will make you squint and will highlight any wrinkles! Softer light will be more flattering.

- Always relax your hands and arms; have them softly draped or gently curved, for a more graceful pose.

- Keep hair sexily tousled; this is very flattering in nude portraits, softening the face (and helping to conceal any lines on your neck!).

- Elevate your face; it's always flattering to be shot from above. Pose sitting down, looking up to the camera, lifting your chin up. This will let the light fall on your face, giving you amazing cheekbones!

- Do smile directly at the camera; this will show how relaxed and confident you are in your body.

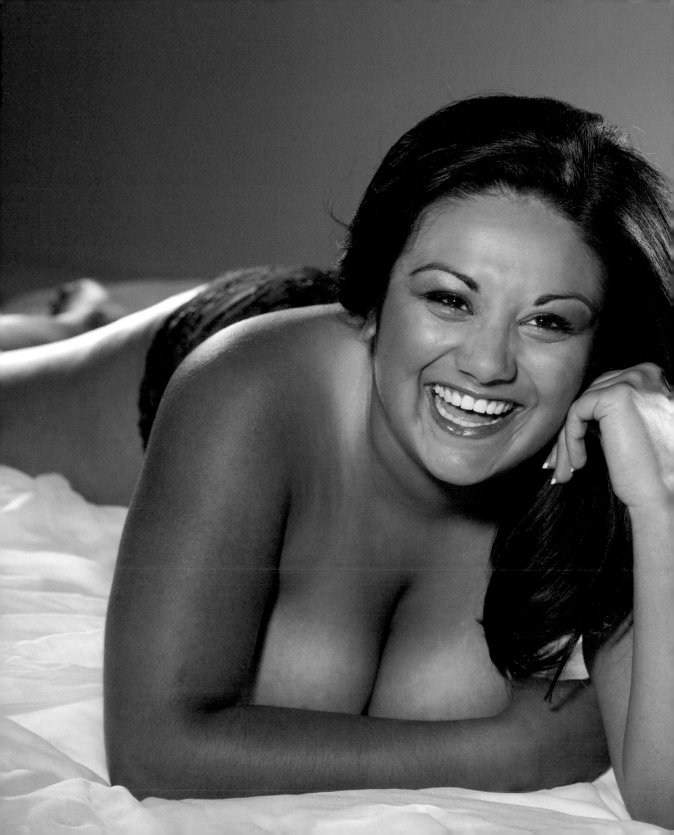

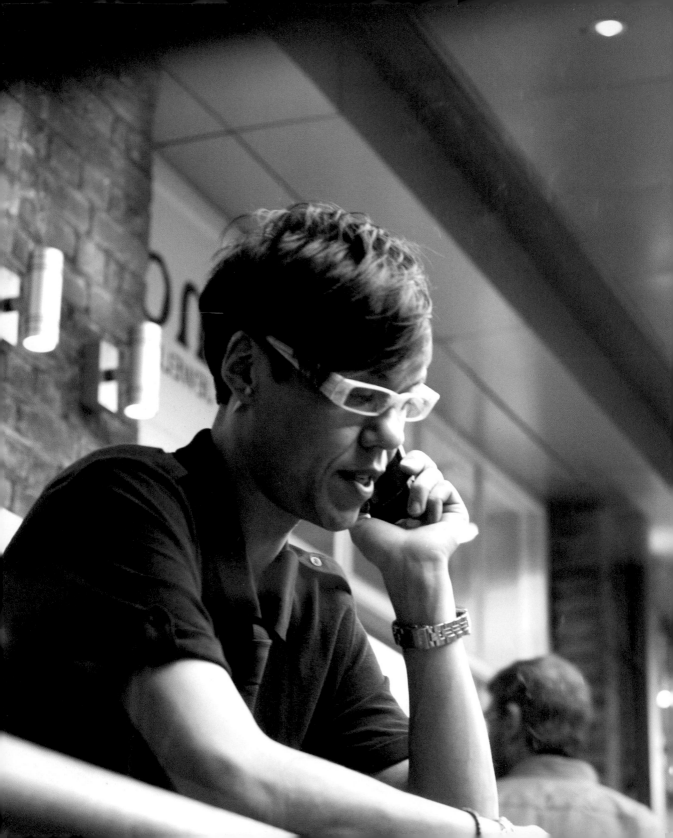

Acknowledgements

A massive thank you to everybody who has made this book possible. I've loved every minute of it. Special thanks go particularly to:

My absolutely amazing family who have believed in me even when I didn't: John Tung Shing, Myra, Oilen, Kwoklyn, Lisa, Maya Lily and Lola Rose.

'Lainey V' for such friendship, without you nothing is possible! 'Baby' for teaching me so much about life, love and laughter, and 'Meneh' for years of confidence, guidance and debauchery.

My agent Carol Hayes (boss bird) whose unflinching support from the very beginning has made it all possible, my assistant Tony Hortel (Spanish bird) and his legendary patience, especially when I was wrong, and Diana and Ian for making me 'keep it real!'.

To everybody at Maverick Television and Channel 4 who has been involved with the show, particularly Colette Foster (scary bird), Victoria Phelan (organized bird) for not leaving that office since Feb '06, Jane Galpin (manic bird), Electra (fashion bird), Sue Murphy and Philippa Ransford. It's been fabulous, you're all fabulous and fabulous is just simply fabulous!

To Angela Buttolph (trendy bird) for helping me write this book. Honey, I would have been lost without you – one day I want to grow up and be you!

To Mike Owen and his team for his amazing photography and to his agent Nigel Barnes for making it possible.

To David Leahy for the fabulous reportage photography at Harriet's Muse, off Carnaby Street. Thanks also to the lovely Cheryl, Craig and Michelle for letting us pitch up pre-London fashion week. You were brilliant.

To everybody at HarperCollins Publishers, particularly designer extraordinaire Jacqui Caulton (vampy bird), my editors Sally Potter and Susanna Abbott (posh bird), my publicist Laura Summers and Eve Fernandez in marketing.

To Rigby & Peller, particularly my second Mum, June Kenton, for all their help with the underwear and swimwear.

To Mark Lesbirel at RDF for bringing us all together.

To the lovely Mary-Ann Ochota, Daisy Idwal Jones, Anne-Marie Barretto and Pippa Jeffreys who modelled for the photographs in this book. Thanks also to my girls from the first series – the original Gok-ettes ... You go girlfriends!

Lastly... to all the women out there who stand up and are proud to be you! What an inspiration!

Directory

Please contact the following suppliers for further information on the clothes featured in this book.

Marks & Spencer – 0845 3021234
Zara – 020 7534 9500
House of Fraser – 020 7936 2000
French Connection – 020 7493 3124
Coast – 01865 881986
Dorothy Perkins – 020 7467 8971
Evans – 020 7467 8971
Topshop – 020 7467 8971
Next – 0845 4567808
Shush – 01506 460250

All underwear and swimwear from Rigby & Peller – 0845 076 5545

Special thanks also to Debenhams for all of their support.